Praise for *AIDS Orphans Rising*

"I personally know Sister Mary Elizabeth and totally endorse her and her book. She is coming from her heart and sincerely wants to make a difference in the world. This book is a treasure and a guide."

—Joe Vitale, author of *The Key*, costar in *The Secret*

"Sr. Mary Elizabeth has gifted us with a marvelous book! Her scientific study on the crisis of AIDS in children of underdeveloped countries is written in a compassionate, caring manner that deeply touches and moves the heart of the reader. It is a book that will affect you profoundly. I am proud and honored to commend this outstanding work."

—Sister Mary De Bacco, M.P.F., Superior General

"Here is a realistic, meticulously-researched look at the problems faced by the millions of AIDS orphans in Africa, and the people who are attempting to care for them.

But even more, this is a story of the transcendence of the human spirit, as we learn about children facing their challenges with incredible resilience, determination, and yes - even joy. We in the west must not give up on them, because they are certainly not giving up on themselves."

—Jillian C. Wheeler, CEO, author, philanthropist

"This book is an inspiring gem of human caring for human. Particularly, the last chapter is beautiful and inspiring. It is very clearly written, and for the ordinary reader, and yet it is a fully documented scholarly work."

—Bob Rich, PhD, author *Cancer: A Personal Challenge*

AIDS ORPHANS RISING

WHAT YOU SHOULD KNOW AND
WHAT YOU CAN DO TO HELP THEM SUCCEED

Sister Mary Elizabeth Lloyd, M.P.F, Ed.D.

www.AIDSOrphansRising.org

Library of Congress Cataloging-in-Publication Data

Lloyd, Mary Elizabeth.
AIDS orphans rising : what you should know and what you can do to help them succeed / Sister Mary Elizabeth Lloyd.
p. cm.
Includes bibliographical references and index.
ISBN-13: 978-1-932690-47-7 (trade paper : alk. paper)
ISBN-10: 1-932690-47-6 (trade paper : alk. paper)
1. AIDS (Disease)--Social aspects. 2. Children of AIDS patients. 3. Orphans. 4. Youth-headed households. I. Title.
RA643.8.L66 2008
362.196'9792--dc22

2007047767

Published by:
Loving Healing Press
5145 Pontiac Trail
Ann Arbor, MI 48105
USA

http://www.LovingHealing.com or
info@LovingHealing.com
Fax +1 734 663 6861

Loving Healing Press

Table of Contents

Table of Figures

100% of all profits from this book will go to help the Child Headed Households.

Donations to help may be sent c/o
Religious Teachers Filippini Mission Fund
455 Western Ave.
Morristown, NJ 07960

And they are tax deductible!

This book has been written with the intention to inform as many people as possible about the situation of the AIDS orphans and their Child Headed Households. I have made a great effort to recognize everyone whose works have been used to help explain this cause. Should you feel I have slighted you or any group please write to me, and I will make the proper insertions. srmelloyd@gmail.com

How the Book Began

Retrieving my suitcase from the hallway, I heard a faint knock at the door. Upon opening it, I found two little boys. One said, "My name is Moses," and the other, in a very frail manner said, "I'm Abraham." Biblical names, was my first thought!

Moses, who looked about 9 years old, began by saying that they were students in our school, and could we help them? Their older sister had left them this morning right after their older brother, just released from prison, had taken all their food and money!

This was some story for me to digest after just having arrived in Adigrat, Ethiopia from the United States. I called one of the Sisters, and she said she would give them some food now, and later we would go to visit with them. She told me they had lost their parents to HIV/AIDS. She was quick to add, "There are about 600 children like this in town."

We, the Religious Teachers Filippini, have been helping the women and children of the Tigray Region of Ethiopia and Eritrea to succeed in life through our elementary schools and women promotion centers for more than 30 years. We have seen the effects of wars and famines, but never, never have we experienced anything like this!

Later that afternoon, we walked over to see how the boys were doing. Until today, Sister explained, they were "on the rise." The two boys were doing well in our elementary school. Abraham (see pic I-1), was being treated by the doctor for his tuberculosis of the bone, but able to go to school each day. The older sister was in our program where she was working for her elementary school diploma and also receiving training in running a knitting machine. She was on her way to one day having her own business. Like so many of the orphans they are working so hard to have a great life one day.

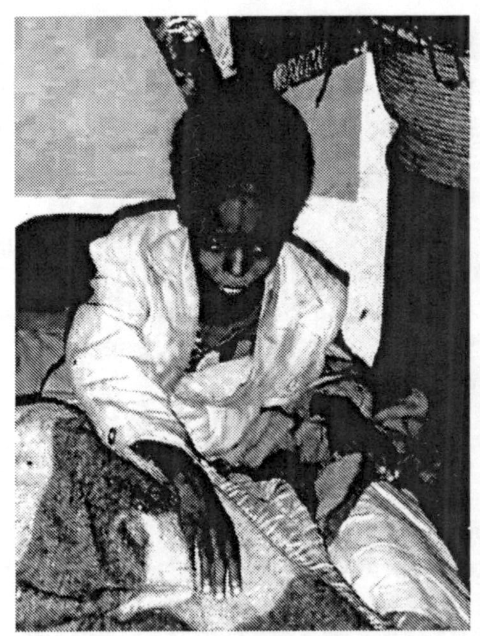

Pic. I-1: Abraham alone again with TB of the bone

This small family was my introduction to the little known phenomenon of Child Headed Households (CHH), one of which is now formed every 14 seconds. The growing phenomenon of CHH scraping for survival shows the determination of the remnants of families to stay together, living off the kindness of strangers and the scant attention of social workers. Alienated by the stigma of parents who have died of AIDS, the orphan families "burdened beyond their years", who nonetheless carry on working and attending school.[1] These children are Africa's chance to break the cycle of poverty that has held a grip on the continent for centuries. With help from people who believe in them and a good education, these children, with their courage and perseverance, will show us all what good can be accomplished. My hope is that this book will help you to understand the plight of these children, to help them, succeed now.

How to read this book

The order in which you read the chapters in this book is not important to the understanding of the information. Check the Table of Contents and go to the part that interests you most. The book is well documented for those interested in further study of this situation.

Be sure not only to read these pages but to *take action today* on any of the ideas you find at the end of each chapter that tell you what you can do now to help these orphans!

Introduction

AIDS Orphans Rising will introduce you to children orphaned by AIDS, and struggling to keep their family together. Most policy guidelines for children portray them as victims, dependent and powerless. Little attention has been given to the positive aspects of these children's behavior and how they have been able to take control of their lives. In this book you will see brothers and sisters from one to eighteen years of age fighting all the odds to stay together. It is not a sad story. For them this is life; they see it all around them and they see those who get up and go on to survive. It is a tremendous story of courage, of children willing to forgo education, and their childhood itself for the sake of their family. This is the story of children who with a little help and love will grow up to be fine citizens of the 21st Century.

Statistics from around the world have been included so you see the vastness of this problem and that it might touch your heart to go out of your way to help these children. We who have had a wonderful childhood, brought up by loving and protective parents, have the knowledge and wherewithal to reach out to these children. And those of you reading who perhaps did not have the best parents in the world at least had hugs and healthcare and school, something these children may never receive without your help.

Reading this work will be beneficial to you, as many of us know little of the plight or successes of these children. Yes, television and concerts are great at telling you there is an AIDS crisis and there are orphans. You see them poor and hungry and helpless in a quick glance, but this work will allow you to see more closely not just what these children are up against, but how they can succeed and how you can make a difference in their lives.

Many people believe HIV infection levels are exaggerated. Of the over 1 billion people aged 15-24 worldwide, some 10 million are living with HIV. Ten percent of the 42

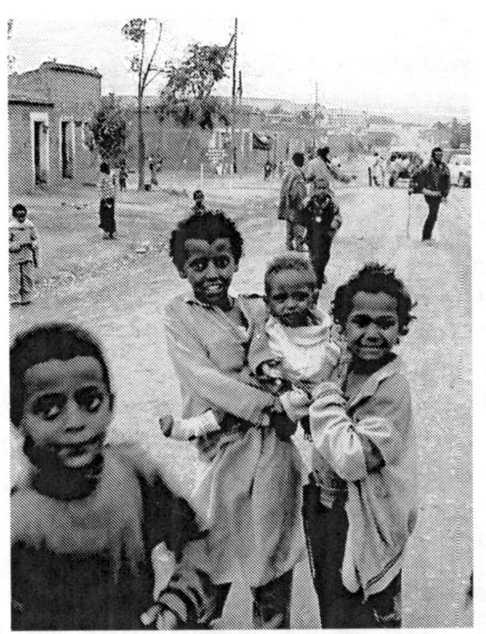

Pic. I-2: A young CHH doing their best

million people living with HIV are children under 18 years of age. Every day, an estimated 6,000 youth are infected with the virus.

Can you visualize how quickly the virus can spread? Try this quick exercise. Take a sheet of paper, and ask yourself this question: How many times will I need to fold the sheet before it is 250 pages thick? Actually, you only need to fold it eight times! And so, too, does the HIV/AIDS virus spread. In 2001, Emma Guest in her book on the AIDS orphan crisis stated, "The sheer numbers of orphans now are something that's so morally reprehensible that people are taking note. Children inspire guilt!"[2] The geometric progression continues at greater speed among populations affected by AIDS. And as the number of infected adults rises, so too does the number of AIDS orphans increase. A new Child Headed Household is formed every 14 seconds![3] Of the millions of women infected with AIDS, only a third will transmit the virus to their babies, and fewer than one in ten babies will be infected.[4] Very few of these men and women will have access to life-extending drugs. Soon, all of the mothers and fathers will die, leaving behind not only their babies but also those babies' siblings, all of the children now orphans.

The UN publication *Children on the Brink*[5] provides the broadest and most comprehensive statistics yet on the historical, current, and projected number of children orphaned by HIV/AIDS.

As you read the chart below, your eyes see such large numbers, the MEGO (*my eyes glaze over*) effect takes place. It is impossible for the human mind to grasp the enormity of the tragedy. We are talking of more than 16 Million children in just one year who have no mother or father!

Country	Children Orphaned
India	3,700,000
China	2,300,000
Nigeria	870,000
Indonesia	620,000
Bangladesh	540,000
Pakistan	540,000
Congo, Dem Rep.	480,000
Ethiopia	470,000
Brazil	470,000
Total	9,990,000
Total Orphans in all regions of the World	16,100,000

Within the topic of AIDS orphans, there are so many diverse areas that need help, but this book will not be about street kids living alone, not about orphans with AIDS but about healthy brothers and sisters who have lost their parents from AIDS, that want to keep together as a family.

Peter McDermot, head of UNICEF's HIV/AIDS department in Zambia, warns that "the biggest danger when you're portraying suffering is the pornography of depiction. We have to be careful we're not promoting just another black child deserving charity. We have to portray the positives. It's easy to show yet another African failure, whereas in fact the amount of good work going on is unbelievable.

The vast majority of orphans in this country are already being looked after by communities, without any external assistance."[6]

How these children are helped will directly influence the kind of adults they become, the country they inherit, and the world. These are the next generation of voters, taxpayers and leaders, and parents. If we fail to provide for the spiritual, moral, emotional, psychological and physical needs of these children, not only will we have failed them personally, but one can only imagine the chaos that will descend upon us and future generations, affecting all the countries of the world for many years to come. Historians one hundred years from now will regard the HIV/AIDS epidemic as a fundamental determinant for most of the history of the 21st century.[7]

1 What is a Child Headed Household?

Every 14 seconds a Child Headed Household is formed.[1] But what exactly is a Child Headed Household? In this picture you see children who have survived the death of their parents from AIDS, little brothers and sisters struggling to stay alive and remain together as a family. A Child Headed Household is defined as a family unit in which the oldest person residing in the household is under the age of eighteen. Since both parents have died, these children are often referred to in literature as *double orphans*[2]. This is not a new phenomenon to history, but in previous years, most Child Headed Households (from now on referred to as CHH) came about because the parents had died from war. Today there are still CHH being formed by the tragedy of war, but half of all CHH are formed because the parents have died from HIV/AIDS. And there are thousands of "social orphans", i.e., children who have been taken in by family or community members because their parents are unable to care for them due to illness or other circumstances.[3] Orphans of war cry and can tell their story over and over. Children orphaned by AIDS cry, mostly silently behind closed doors. They have no one to tell their story to, and now there are so many that no one wants to know the details, they all know the sickness and the horrible agonizing death of these poor people[4].

Traditional coping mechanisms are being threatened as communities are overwhelmed with the scale of the problem. These are children who watch their parents die long and agonizing deaths; who watch the mortifying process of physical decline; who observe the family struggling and disintegrating before their eyes; who watch the household food security wither away; who watch the tiny income dis-

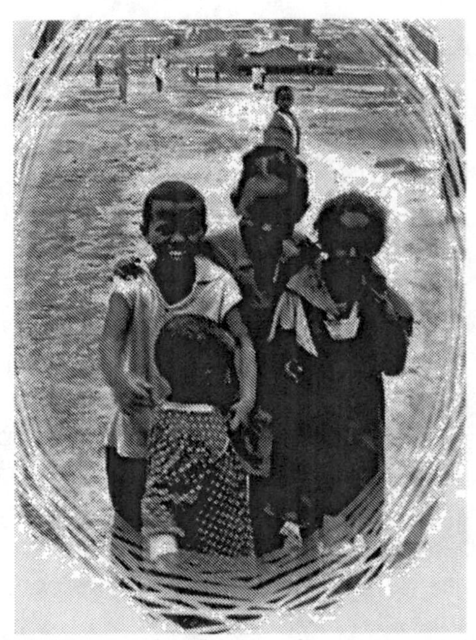

Pic. 1-1: A young family struggling to stay together

appear; who plead for medicines for their mothers and can't get them; who are forced to leave school; who feel forlorn, terrified and abandoned when death claims its victims, victims whom the children loved as only children can love.[5]

"The worst is yet to come," warns a report issued by the UN Children's Fund. The data from UNICEF, UNAIDS and USAID indicates that in sub-Saharan Africa, 14 million children have been orphaned by AIDS—a number higher than the total number of boys and girls under 18 years-old in Canada, Norway, Sweden, Denmark and Ireland combined. That figure is expected to reach 18 million by 2010.

These children, 50 per cent of whom are 10 to14 years old, will be left without critical guidance, protection and support[6]. The problem is overwhelming and the need is immense, but we can help them.

Three quarters of all CHH are led by girls. Picture 1-2 shows a CHH led by an 11 year old girl who is trying to raise her 2 younger sisters, her 2 younger brothers, and go to school. There are usually three to eight children per household, and these orphaned children try to stick together as much as possible. One study of CHHs in Rakai, Uganda, showed that the number of orphans who had lost both parents and were living on their own increased from 4.4% of all orphans from 1985 to 1989 to an incredible 60% between 1995 and 1999.[7] Their right to support, and to remain in charge of their lives without fear of being split up or sent away, must be protected.[8]

These children encounter frequent illnesses and experience high mortality rates, because many of them are less than five years of age. Most of them are exposed to a poor environment, malnutrition, and lack of medical attention, which further compromises their quality of life. Dr. M.A. Ayieko of the United Nations Development Program[9] has documented that when a husband dies of AIDS in a family, the mother is also often living with HIV/AIDS and dies shortly thereafter, leaving the children as orphans. Even if they are aware of their terminal illness, few parents attempt to make any alternative living arrangements for their children before their death. Many believe the grandparents or extended family members will provide for the children. Most of the dying parents are usually so sick and living in such terrible conditions that they don't have the strength or wherewithal to provide for the future of their children.

Left alone, the children must provide for themselves. They often resort to begging for money for food and clothing. Some girls resort to prostitution to raise money.[10] Fetching water, cooking and cleaning are all tasks that are shared among the children. Such children face threats to their survival[11] and often threats to their security. They have the emotional needs common to children everywhere, but they also have special needs, such as palliative care and something often most of these will never receive: bereavement counseling.[12]

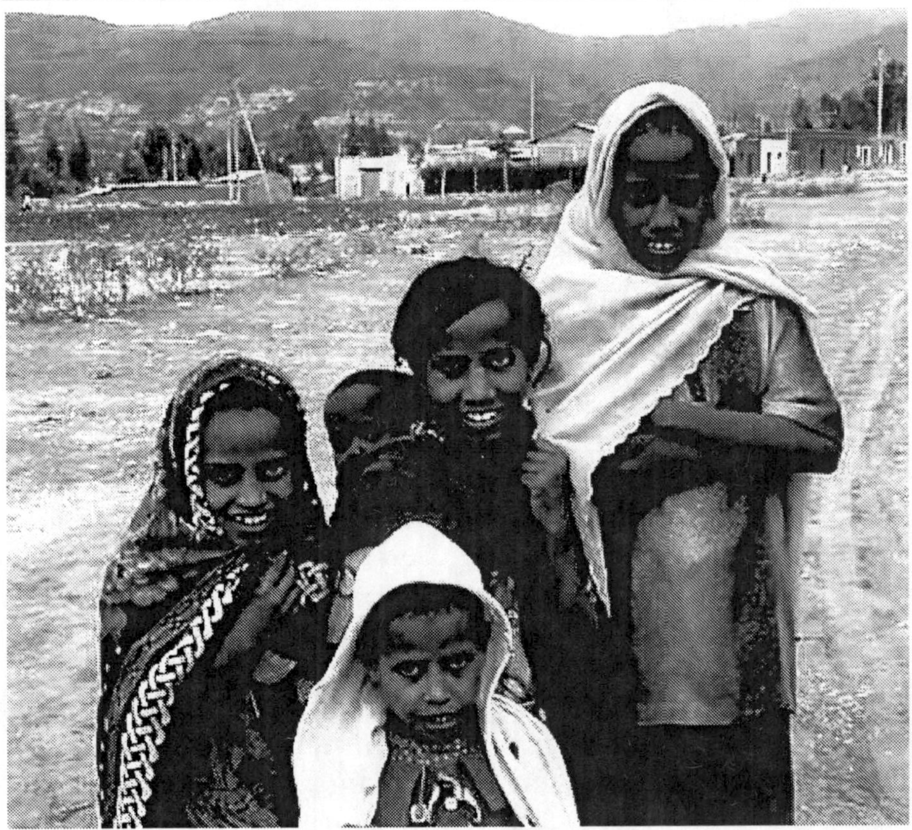

Pic. 1-2: Every 14 seconds a little family like this is formed!

Adolescents from 11 to 15 years of age are in a crucial stage of their social development process, and they need parental guidance. These youth, like the older boy holding his brother in Pic. 1-3, are treated as young adults and expected to behave as mature adults with families. As much as they try to work and provide some leadership for their brothers and sisters, they are still children. They need guidance, time and a chance to be children, to be teenagers and to experience this important stage of human development. The death of a father deprives children of male authority, a status symbol in many communities. But the subsequent death of a mother further deprives the children of crucial emotional and mental security as well.

According to a report[13] by the Christian-based World Vision, CHH are deprived of love, security, a sense of belonging, acceptance and care. They have no one to turn to and live in very difficult circumstances, without the basic necessities of life. They are usually exploited or taken advantage of, hence the loss of trust in the society that is supposed to protect them. Most of the property left behind by their parents has been taken away by relatives or neighbors. Children in such conditions are deprived of their childhood and the opportunity to go to school. Economic hardships lead them to look for means of subsistence that increase their vulnerability to HIV infection, substance abuse, child labor, sex work and delinquency. The International Community virtually ignored the issue of AIDS orphans between 1991-97. "The fear was that it was a charity issue," said Susan Hunter (formerly of UNICEF & USAID) while speaking at the first conference on AIDS orphans in South Africa in 1998, "…there was no way the North could support all the orphans in the South, so none of the donors or international agencies really wanted to put effort into it. They decided instead to put effort into AIDS prevention. There was a time when we believed that we could stop the epidemic."[14]

The determination of the remnants of these families to stay together was the motivation behind the writing of this book. The CHH can be an emerging positive coping mechanism for affected communities. The term itself, Child Headed Household, emphasizes the resilience and power of children heading families living under these circumstances.

We cannot view these children as helpless! That would send a message to them that their own efforts to cope are not seen as legitimate, or indeed even recognized at all. This lack of acknowledgement of children's own strategies can undermine their ability to act on their situation. It is vital to recognize that children's own perspectives on adversity, and the strategies they employ for their own protection, are critical to coping and resilience.[15]

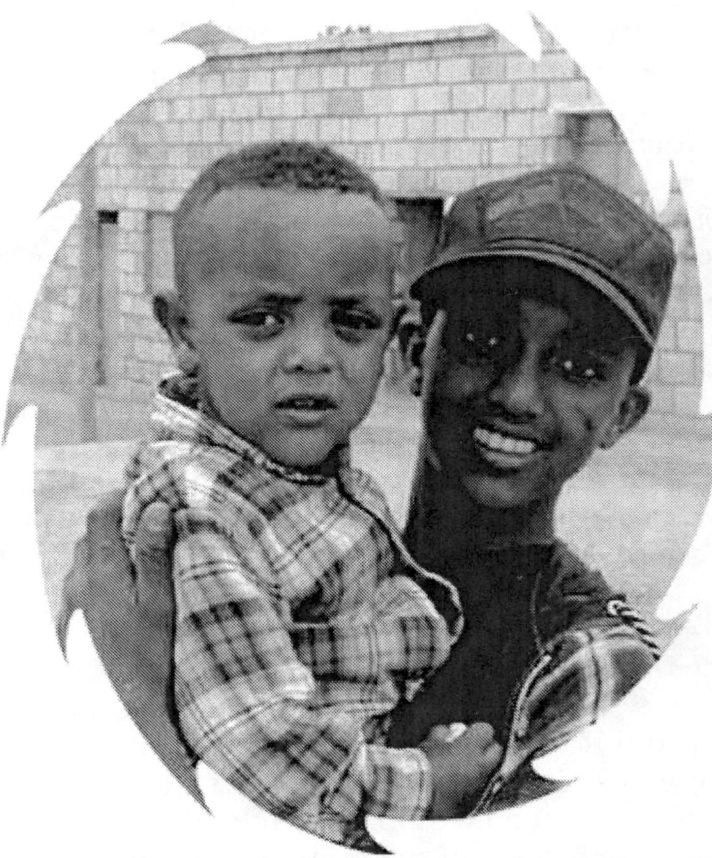

Pic. 1-3: Teens must take on the role of the adults in this world

The following chapters will explain how these children live, eat, study, work, play and laugh and survive despite all odds, and what you can do to help them succeed.

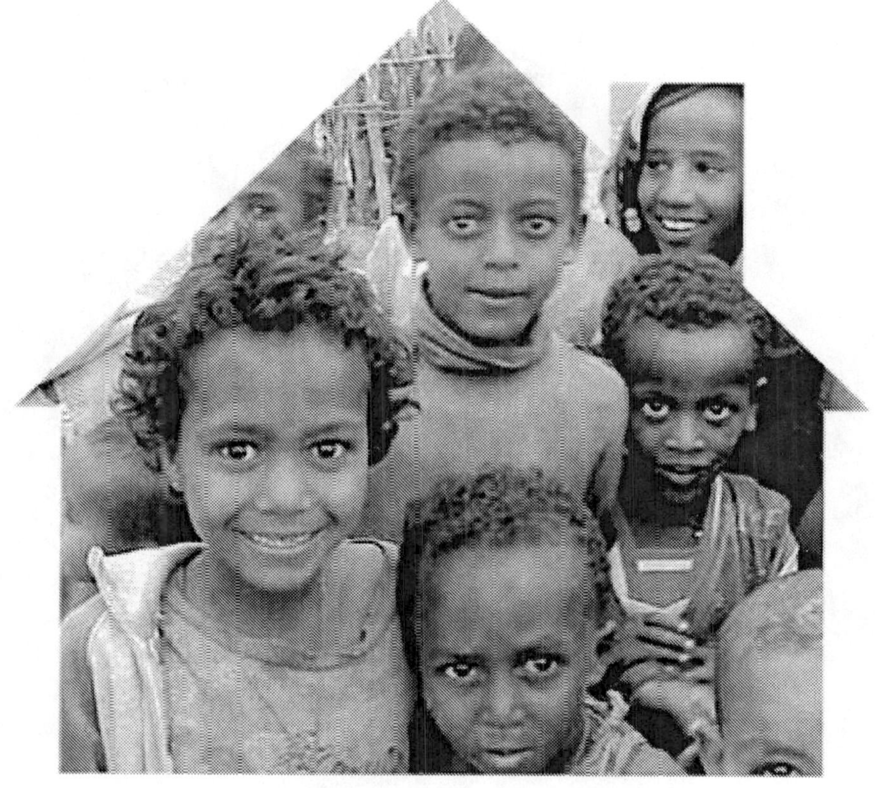

Pic. 1-4: So many need your help

What You Can Do To Help Now!

- Say a quick prayer for these children and all who are helping them.
- Continue reading this book to learn more; go to the suggested web sites for more information.
- Send a check or donate online to an organization that helps CHH.
- Send an email to all in your address book explaining the plight of these children.

2 Where Do They Live?

With more than 13 million children under the age of 15 orphaned by HIV/AIDS, where are they all living? The girl shown in Pic. 2-1 lives under the blue tarp with her little brother seen on her back. Many, many CHH live in homes of plastic sheeting. Often the children huddle together near the train tracks. One child explained, "When you live near the train tracks, you don't hear the trains go by in the middle of the night no matter how loud they are!" They sleep in caves and huddle with animals for warmth. Those who have found a shelter often sleep on bare floors, many with no blankets. Those that have a bed, often have no mattress. They live in a one-room house; food is scarce, and they sleep on a flour sack resting on the cement floor. There is no running water, and no electricity. No bathrooms, no showers. Check your sewer! Type in "children living in sewers" into Google. You will get more than 2,000,000 hits! These are not all orphans of AIDS, but many homeless children in need of help. 15,000 children live this way in Mexico City, but there may be three times more.[1]

Some children, very few in number, fortunately have been left by their deceased parents a small, but safe and secure house in relatively good condition where they can continue to live. Usually it is a typical concrete block house with metal-framed windows, metal roof, and a dung floor. There are three rooms, a kitchen, sitting room and bedroom. They have a pit latrine away from the house on a corner of their property.

Often when the last parent dies at home, the orphans move from their parents' house to live with grandparents or move in with uncles and aunts. Grandparents and other relatives have absorbed some of the responsibility

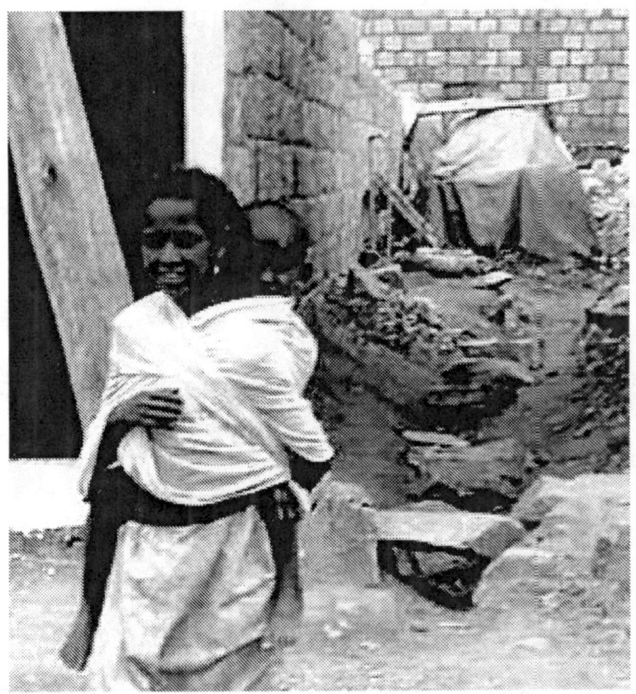

Pic. 2-1: Sleeping under the blue tarp is better than the street

for caring for AIDS orphans, but family networks are sagging under the weight of the epidemic. Many move in with relatives whose desperate poverty only becomes worse with more mouths to feed.

Most especially when a mother dies of AIDS, orphaned children often go to live with a grandmother, a practice referred to as 'skip-generation parenting'.[2] Orphans are often cared for by grandparents because there is no other relative willing or able to look after the children. Grandparent-headed orphan households are becoming increasingly common as a result of AIDS. For example in Zimbabwe, 125 out of 292 orphan households (43%) were headed by grandparents; in Kenya, 41 out of 152 (27%) were grandparent-headed. Even in New York, 25 out of 43 maternal orphans (58%) lived with a grandmother. Some of the most vulnerable orphans are children of single mothers, especially if the mother was a prostitute.

When a single mother becomes sick or dies, her children may be left in the care of grandparents. Because such orphans are from single-parent households, they may be neglected by other relatives who refuse to provide any support to the children because they consider them illegitimate.[3] All too often, a grandparent is already caring for grandchildren from three or four families. The responsibility for orphan care is shifting increasingly to grandmothers who often single-handedly care for 10 to 15 orphans.[4]Many women infected by HIV migrate back to their maternal homes[5] after their husbands have died and they are in the later stages of their illness. Their hope is that the children will find a male authority such as a grandfather or uncle, and social and emotional security with her family. When the mothers eventually die, such orphans are twice disadvantaged by a second trauma of parental death and adjusting to unfamiliar relatives in a foreign place.

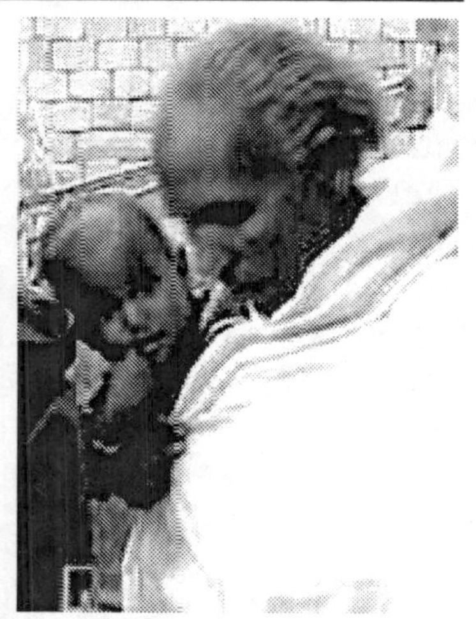

Pic. 2-2: Grandmothers are burdened beyond belief

A Kenyan study found that whereas families living below the poverty line tended to foster children, wealthier relatives, whom one might expect to be more able to foster relatives' children, maintained minimal links with orphans.[6]

Many of these children then move again to new localities to live with relatives and family friends. Often in situations where many sleep in the same hut or a single room, the young girls are abused by the men. This is often the reason many women prefer not to accept the orphan daughters of their own family. Some run away[7] in an effort to find a more suitable living arrangement for themselves. When both parents have died and no relatives accept the children, the CHH usually leave their hometown or village and head to a large city. When they arrive in the cities, the CHH often end up living on the streets and are at extremely high risk of exploitation and HIV infection. Nowhere are the problems more acute than in KwaZulu Natal (KZN), South Africa, an area with the highest rates of HIV/AIDS infection and orphanhood in the whole country. Durban attracts the highest number of street children of any city in Southern Africa.[8]

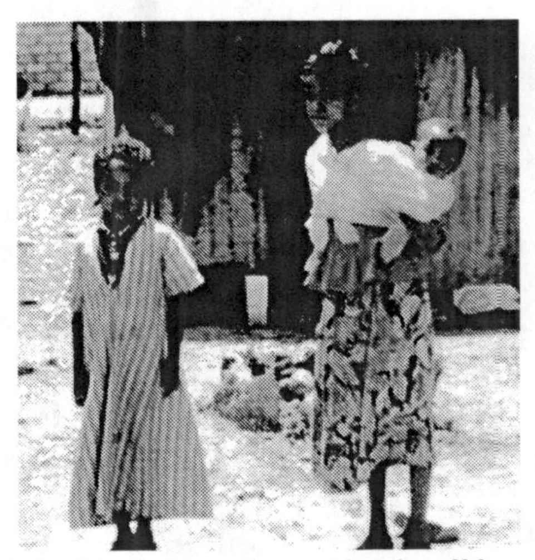

Pic. 2-3: Sick of abuse, these girls take off for town

In nearly every sub-Saharan country, extended families have assumed responsibility for more than 90 per cent of orphaned children. But this traditional support system is under severe pressure—and in many instances has already been overwhelmed, increasingly impoverished and rendered unable to provide adequate care for children. Most worryingly, it is precisely those countries that will see the largest increase in orphans over the coming years where the extended family is already most stretched by caring for orphans.[9]

> During her mother's illness, her mother would request her every night to heat water on the open fire and to wash her mother's feet with the heated water. She knew that her mother was very sick and needed her, but her mother advised her during her illness to live with an aunt, as she said that Sakhisiwe's older sister would take care of her. She feels guilty that she had left her mother during her mother's last few living days, and that is the reason she claims she misses her mother even more. According to Sakhisiwe, when her mother was alive her mother was able to provide everything and even basics like soap to bathe with. Currently there are days when not even soap is available to either bathe or wash their clothes with. She trusted that her mother would provide everything that she needed although currently her grandmother provides for them if and when money is available. She remembers her mother especially when she is provoked while playing with other children. Sakhisiwe Myeni is a 12 year old grade four schoolgirl. 10

One study in Blantyre, Malawi, found that, of the 65 orphans they interviewed, 22 had experienced multiple migrations, some as many as five.[11] Many AIDS-affected children in southern Africa engage in migration when household members fall sick or die from AIDS, or because they are sent to assist relatives. Despite this, little attention has been paid to the consequences of these movements for children's lives. Research, conducted in Lesotho and Malawi, reveals that children sent to live with kin commonly move over long distances and between urban and rural areas. They are generally not consulted or informed about these migrations and face a range of associated difficulties, particularly with integrating into new families and communities. Severed family ties exacerbate the difficulties faced by children who end up in institutions or on the streets.

This paper advocates that policy approaches for those affected by AIDS should be children-centered and take into account the implications of migration at three levels.[12] First, many of the difficulties children face could be overcome if they were familiar with the place and people they were moving to. Second, children would be better able to cope with new situations if they were included in family discussions with decision-makers regarding their migration preferences. Third, maintaining ties with kin would ensure that children do not become distanced from their family and cultural heritage, which is essential for post-institutional support.

The fact that orphans are now being fostered by maternal rather than paternal relatives, especially in peri-urban areas, is symptomatic of the decline of traditional extended family practices.[13] Most often when the last parent dies, the extended family, if unable to take care of the orphans, will stay away from them. This is extremely painful for the children and they can't understand why and often put the blame on themselves. Psychological help is also greatly needed for these children, but it is highly unlikely that they will receive it at this present moment. Frequently the children may desire to stay together as a family group rather than be split up between various relatives, or wish to stay living at their own residence in familiar surroundings, rather than change school, friends, home and neighborhood. They may resist attempts of relatives to foster them in the relative's household, fearing maltreatment or because the relative only agrees to foster younger siblings. The main reasons children say they prefer not to live with extended family members are:

- Most of their relatives are very poor and financially unable to support them or are already supporting large extended family members
- They do not want verbal abuse
- They do not want to be exploited for work
- They want to continue their schooling

- They feel that they are better off on their own.

In leaving their home, they leave behind any property that might have been rightfully theirs.[14] In many countries, the inheritance practices are that the paternal relatives receive any property left after the death of their son.[15] Unscrupulous relatives take the land but refuse to take the orphans, pushing them out of the extended family safety net. The children would have to fight to retain their access to land as neighbors and opportunists seek to take advantage of the situation. Most are too young, or so saddened by their loss they pack up the younger children and leave all behind and head to another area. Tragically, orphans who lack the support of relatives remain on their own to fend for themselves. Imagine you are nine years old, with three younger brothers and sisters, and you suddenly have no place to live and no source of income. Here is the home of Esther, Moses and Daniel (see Pic. 2-3). You are right; there is no home in this picture! They have been sleeping near that back rock wall. When her parents died in 2004, nine-year-old Esther became head of the household. The Sisters of St. Lucy have taken them into their hostel for the most neglected CHH. The children are together as a family and are given food, clothing, shelter and schooling. At St. Lucy School the girls enter a special program where they learn skills that allow them provide for their siblings. When the boys get bigger, they will enter the Christian Brothers school in town. The Sisters are trying to keep as many of these children together as a family unit as possible.

SOS Children's Villages are committed to bringing up the children in its care to the best of its ability until they are young adults... not just to provide for the children's emotional stability, but also to prepare them thoroughly for independence. Kindergartens, schools and vocational training are an essential part of this.[16]

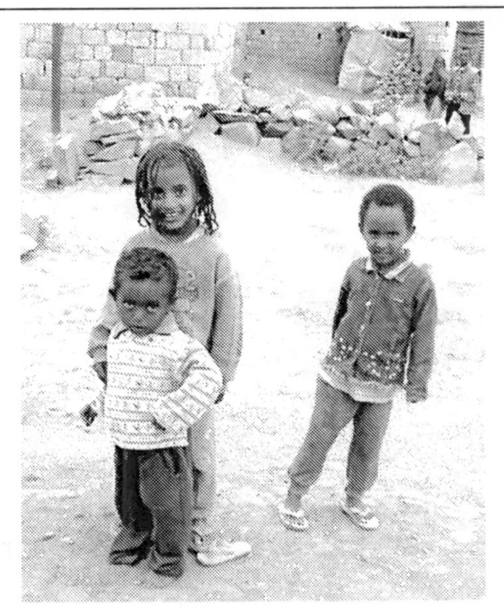

Pic. 2-4: The very young come to live at the convent

Many treaties[17] clearly endorse a policy that orphaned children should not be institutionalized, but should, where at all possible, grow up in some form of family envi ronment. Growing up in communities disrupted by the epidemic, orphans are more likely to cope if they can live in surroundings that are familiar, stable and as nurturing as possible. Many believe that orphans should be cared for in family units[18] through extended family networks, foster families and adoption. UNAIDS states that at the very least, siblings should not be separated. But the extended family[19] or shelters can only serve as part of the solution to mass orphanhood if adequately supported by the state, community and other sectors.

A recent World Vision[20] study of 1,649 CHH found that 95% of these children have no access to healthcare or education, and lack sufficient food, basic household goods, or agricultural necessities.

The UN proposes that adequate housing is a human right.[21] Therefore, the pressure on international governments to provide adequate housing is gaining strength.

Other issues inevitably arise where housing is poor. These issues include lack of food, access to clean water, forced eviction, gender discrimination, poor health, unemployment, low income or no income and urban migration. Children are particularly vulnerable to the impacts of these issues.

Those older children fortunate enough to find some kind of work have to pay a high proportion of their income on rent[22], water, and electricity. This has a direct bearing on how much income is left over to meet their children's food requirements. The children are responsible to build new houses, or repair damage to existing homes. Many Non-Governmental Organizations (NGOs) are helping to pay the children's rent. The Religious Teachers Filippini have a program in Ethiopia where they rent a house for the CHH they find living on the streets. The house rents for $3 a month; it is a 6x4 ft. cement box, no bathroom and no window. In the morning the children come to school to receive nourishment and an education. Habitat for Humanity International, in partnership with Nurturing Orphans of AIDS for Humanity, has secured a $600,000 grant from Comic Relief to build cluster homes for AIDS orphans in 10 communities in Kwazulu-Natal, South Africa.[23]

Indications are that the majority of children orphaned by AIDS at present are not being accommodated through formal placements in alternative care structures. The extended family that would once have absorbed children without parents into communal life can no longer be relied upon to fulfill that function. This has led to the formation of many initiatives in the forms of shelters, safe houses, hostels that have sprung up to help these children.

Julia Sloth-Nielsen, law professor at the University of the Western Cape in South Africa, suggests that the community and home-based care model has reportedly been most successful.[24] These models are based on a children's rights approach, and accept that children orphaned by AIDS face special challenges. These needs, it is said, are often best met in supportive community settings. Community and home-based care models mostly use volunteers as the backbone of a care-giving strategy. Empowering affected children[25] first of all means regarding them as active members rather than just victims. Many children already function as heads of households and as caregivers. They are a vital part of the solution and should be supported in planning and carrying out efforts to lessen the impact of HIV/AIDS in their families and communities.

Despite concern about ethical dilemmas attached to the idea of children staying on their own without parents or adult supervision, it has been observed that it is possible with appropriate support from NGOs and other community support systems for orphans to be nurtured in CHHs.[26]

Strategies and interventions are required to protect all children's rights to adequate shelter, such as by improving housing, clothing and ensuring child friendly environments.[27] Sometimes, adolescents have to make a deathbed promise to take care of young children and keep them together.[28,29] As a result of such promises, adolescents who might otherwise prefer to see the other children placed in foster homes resist reasonable strategies suggested by relatives or child welfare authorities. Community groups can help extended families to cope with the burden of orphans by encouraging the establishment of volunteer-based visiting programs to at risk households and by channeling essential material support to destitute families.

The emergence of households headed by children sometimes as young as 10-12 years old is one of the most distressing consequences of the epidemic. Though it is often assumed that the presence of these households in communities implies that extended family methods of support have broken down, this assumption has not been validated since there have been no previous studies of child-

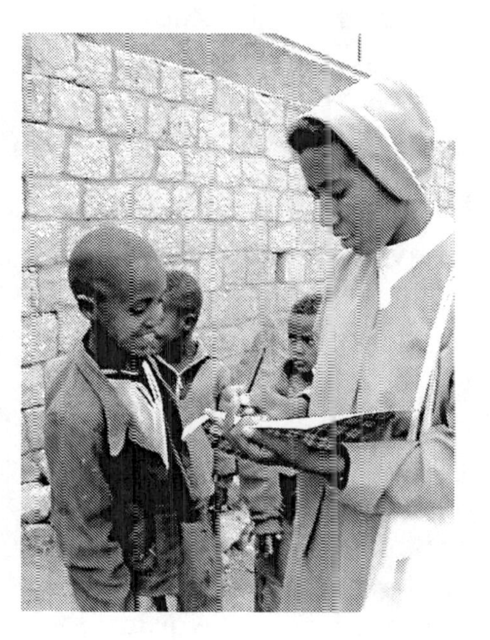

Pic. 2-5: Sister helps these children, who have just arrived in town, find food and lodging, and signs them up in school.

headed households. We may develop appropriate methods of support to children living in especially difficult circumstances through better understanding of existing coping mechanisms.

In a study of 30 households, 88% stated that the relative did not want to care for the children.
The main reason for refusal to take in relatives' children was probably economic. In many cases, aunts and uncles provided material support or regularly visited child-headed households; in some cases it was stated that relatives did not foster children in their own families because they lived nearby and instead had chosen to regularly visit.[30]

These are indications that in many cases, households headed by children or adolescents are a new expression of the extended family's coping mechanism rather than the result of children slipping through the extended family safety net. Thousands of CHH are rising. They are living on their own, going to school, caring for their siblings and on the way to a very good life. Many more can be put on this same great path if given the opportunity. It is up to the common person, you, and me, all of us, to help them. They can change the face of Africa to one of success!

What You Can Do To Help Now!

- Say a prayer right now for these children and all who are helping them.
- Call the local authorities and ask if there are any orphans from AIDS in your area, and where do they and the "street children" sleep?
- Send a check or donate online to an organization that houses CHH, and be sure to indicate you want it to go for housing for the children:
- This is a great opportunity where those of you trained in psychology would be of invaluable service. Give some weeks of your vacation to a group that is helping the CHH. It would make a tremendous difference in their quality of life and in survival.
- Get involved with the local real estate agencies and see what they might do to help.
- Organize or join a group that might go to a country with many CHH and build homes for them: http://www.frank-mckinney.com/caring_house.html
- Take a thermos of hot tea and some sweet rolls early in the morning to where the "street children" live. You will never be the same.
- Send an email to all in your address book explaining the plight of these children and get your friends to help.

3 What Do They Eat?

All children are happy when given food. Despite the sorrow of having lost their parents, these children continue on with a smile. This young girl is preparing dinner for herself and three siblings. Surely at times the sadness overwhelms them, but normally they are out and about searching for food or whatever they need to survive for that day. Many survive off scraps of food they beg from strangers or salvage from garbage areas. Very young girls, 8 or 9 years old, often assume the heavy responsibilities of working in the garden, preparing and serving meals to both younger and older siblings in the households.

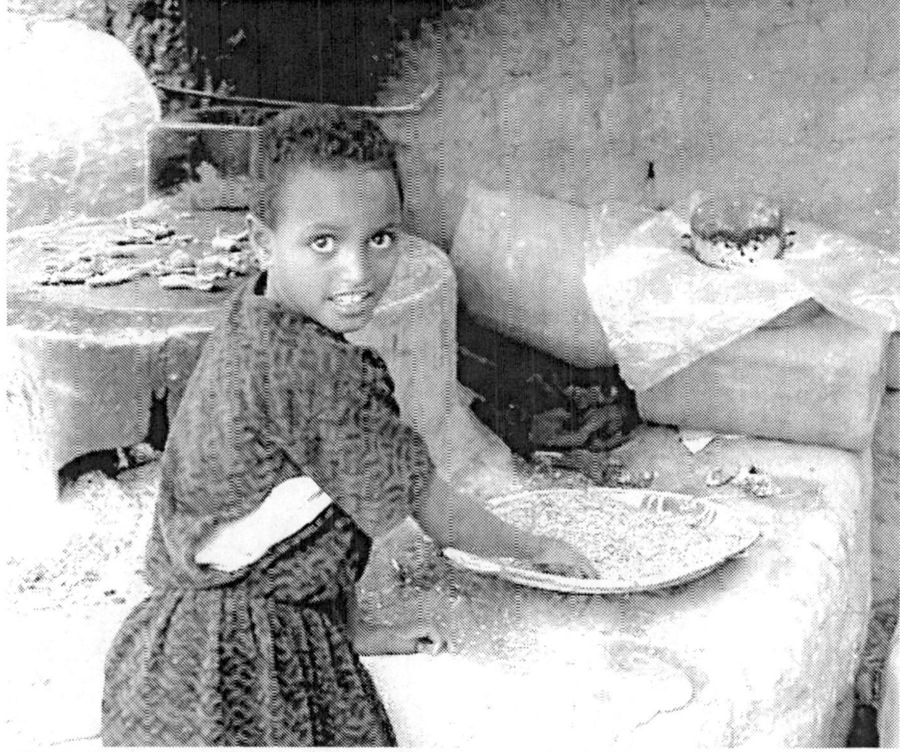

Pic. 3-1: Providing for herself and her siblings, this little one also goes to school fulltime

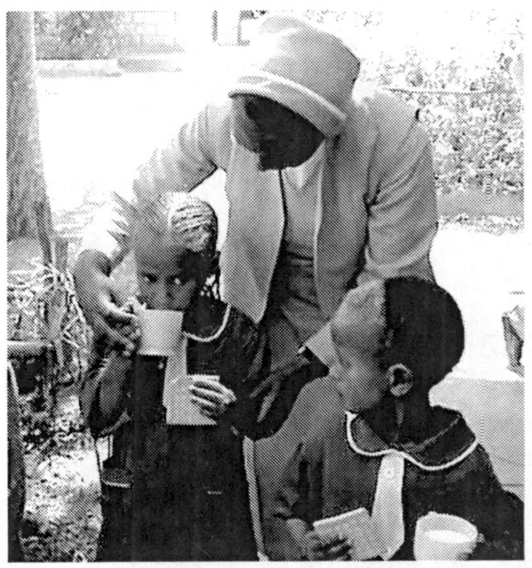

Pic. 3-2: A little scared! The first day of the milk program -- some had never tasted milk before!

These children survive on so little. Most of them I have observed to live on less than 1200 kcal per day. In HIV/AIDS-affected households lacking community support, food consumption can drop by more than 40 per cent, putting children at higher risk of malnutrition and stunting.[1]

The lucky ones attending St. Lucy School in Adigrat, Ethiopia, (pictured above,) receive fortified biscuits and milk. In the near future, the school will implement a hot lunch program. It is good to remember that it was the hot lunch program that ended hunger for children in the USA. Children orphaned by HIV/AIDS face a higher risk of malnutrition and stunting, as seen through sub-national studies of the impact of an adult death on child nutrition. It is difficult to judge from national household surveys the extent to which orphans are becoming malnourished, because the sample sizes of orphans under five are quite small. Research in the United Republic of Tanzania shows that the loss of either parent and the death of other adults in the household will worsen a child's height for age and increase their stunting. Both maternal and paternal orphans are much more likely to be short for their age than non-orphans. In non-poor families, the loss of a parent raises stunting to levels found among children in poor families with living parents. In poor families, orphans raise stunting levels even higher.[3]

> Gordon Gunter of the National School Lunch Program reminds us of our own hunger problems by citing from a **1904** book by Robert Hunter:[2] "The lack of learning among so many poor children is certainly due, to an important extent, to this cause. There must be thousands—very likely sixty or seventy thousand children—in New York City alone who often arrive at school hungry and unfitted to do well the work required. It is utter folly, from the point of view of learning, to have a compulsory school law which compels children, in that weak physical and mental state which results from poverty, to drag themselves to school and to sit at their desks, day in and day out, for several years, learning little or nothing. If it is a matter of principle in democratic America that every child shall be given a certain amount of instruction, let us render it possible for them to receive it, as monarchial countries have done, by making full and adequate provision for the physical needs of the children who come from the homes of poverty."

In Burkino Faso[4] they have had a terrible problem. Cars hit many children as they attempt to cross the road to buy drinking water! Most often they can be seen drinking water from an old rusty leaking pipe. Pictured here are orphans and adults trying to get safe drinking water at a center set up by the World Food Program. Here one finds large canvas bags filled with water, and all are free to come and fill any container they have. The orphans' problem is that they have no container. And the adults push them aside and block them from

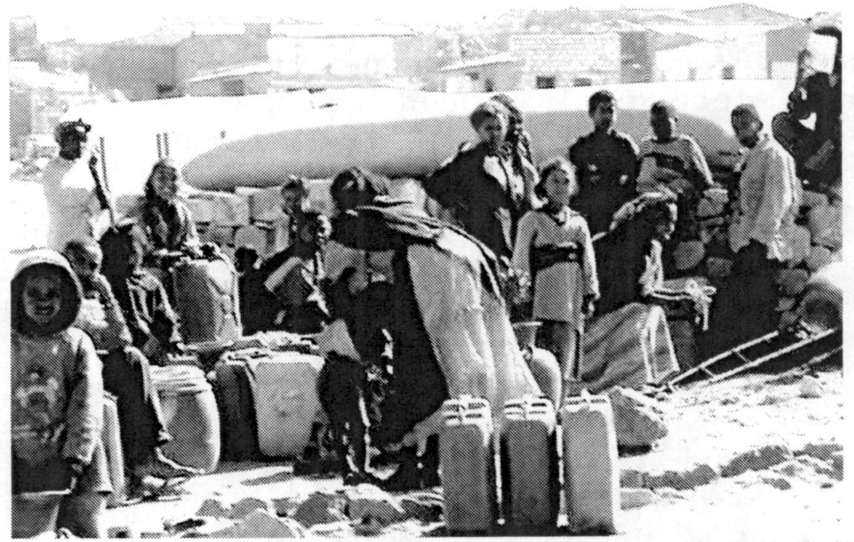

Pic. 3-3: Access to water is very difficult for the orphans, adults control all of it

getting any of the water. "Unfortunately, AIDS orphans end up at the back of feeding lines because they are left to fend for themselves," says Jennifer Abrahamson, of the World Food Program.[5]

Hungry children have a sense for those worse off than themselves. When I gave some bread to this little boy from Ethiopia (see Pic. 3-4), he immediately turned to give it to his dying mother!

Being homeless or surviving in inadequate and insecure housing has a direct bearing on someone's ability to feed himself. Government officials say they do not even have the means to determine how many children need help. In Mozambique, UNICEF projects that by 2010, the country will be home to 1.2-million orphans, 926,000 of them due to AIDS. All of the cash-strapped governments rely on international organizations like WFP to help feed their AIDS orphans. Many fall between the cracks and get no help at all. The food security of these children is a major concern. Lack of adequate land, know-how and water often drive the children from their parents' homes to the cities in search of food.

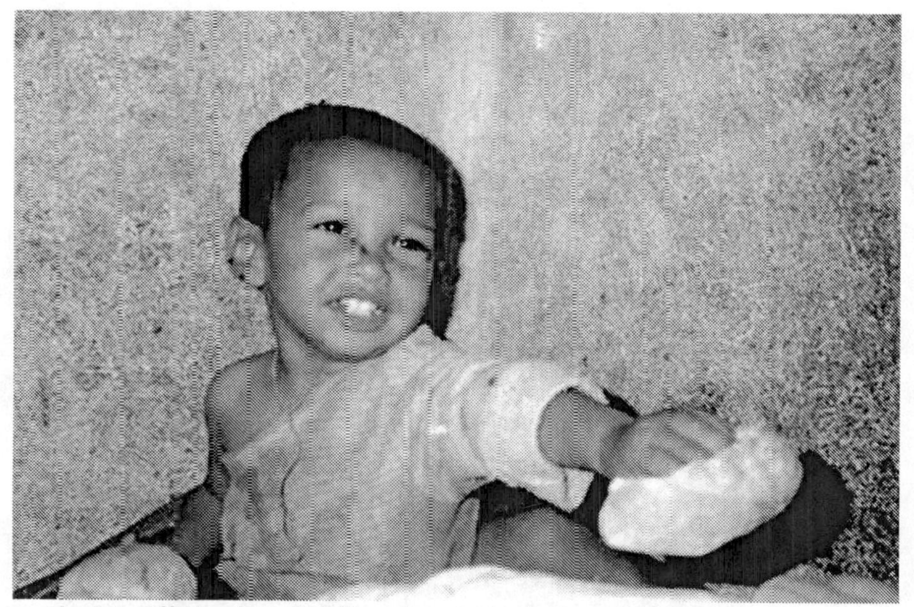

Pic. 3-4: Offering bread to his dying mother before he takes some himself.

These children have arrived at an outdoor shelter where the Sisters provide a good hot meal for the children living alone out under the stars (see Pic. 3-5).

The Farm Orphan Support Trust (FOST) of Zimbabwe in their report, *We Will Bury Ourselves*, say that of the 17 typical CHH interviewed, two of the families specifically mentioned that they regularly go a whole day without eating and often were hungry. Others reported that they were often anxious about getting enough to eat. None of the CHH interviewed regularly ate a balanced diet.[6] The 2003 nutritional survey for Zimbabwe, which weighed and measured nearly 42,000 children, including 1,760 orphans, shows that a higher percentage of orphans are malnourished than non-orphans. The risk is high that these children will never develop to their full physical and intellectual capacity.[7]

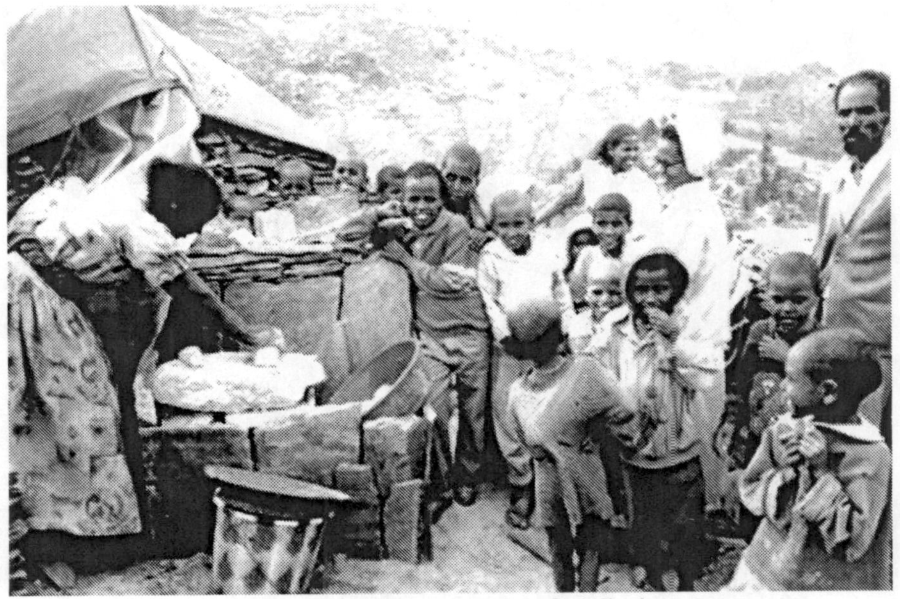

Pic. 3-5: Outdoor kitchens provide for all who come

Many small groups and non-profit organizations are really making heroic attempts at keeping these children alive. You know, today more children die of moderate malnutrition than from severe. In a sense, that is a great sign. The severely malnourished child is being helped. Our next challenge is to end all malnutrition. Many of you have heard the story of a young child walking along the beach picking up starfish and throwing them back in the ocean. An adult comes along and scoffs at him and says, “Why are you doing that? It makes no difference!” The young child replies, “It does to the ones I throw back.” In the same vein Natalie Simione, who runs Liberdade, where 35 AIDS orphans in Mozambique receive three nutritious meals a day, says it best for all of us caring for these children, “We can't save them all, but we will do our best with the ones we can reach.”[8]

What You Can Do To Help Now!

- Find a new dimension in your prayer life as you anonymously and humbly pray for an orphan on the other side of the world who needs your prayers. http://www.prayforanorphan.org/yahoo_ad.htm
- Bring some of the extra food you have to a shelter where there are children.
- Create your own Non-Profit Organization to help feed theses children. To learn how, go to http://www.GrantMeRich.com/classes.htm
- Send a check or donate on line to an organization that feeds CHH, and be sure to indicate you want it to go for food for the children.
- Sign up for AIDS Orphans Rising, which provides updates of the AIDS orphan crisis via email. Join the list now. http://AIDSorphans.blogspot.com
- Send an email to all in your address book explaining the plight of these children and how they can help.
- Sign up for Albina's Action for Orphans, which provides a bi-monthly update of the AIDS Orphans crisis via email. Join the list now. http://www.albinasactionfororphans.org/learn/alerts/alert2.html

4 How Do They Survive?

"Our parents died in 1995. When this happened, our relatives ran away from us. This surprised us because, being our relatives, we thought they would care for us. Our parents had a big farm, but it was taken from us so we had nowhere to grow food. My younger brothers and sisters became beggars; they would walk from house to house asking for food." Africa Recovery, United Nations.[1]

Not uncommonly these days, and contrary to tradition, some relatives may take the property of the deceased relative and leave his or her family to fend for itself. This situation could be avoided if people dying were persuaded to make a written will.

Persistent poverty is seen as the greatest challenge for the CHH. Finding money for food and clothes usually leads the children to beg. Some girls resort to prostitution to raise money. Sex often buys food, but at a high price. In addition to the emotional cost of prostitution, there are rampant sexually transmitted diseases including the risk of acquiring HIV themselves. Children will resort to prostitution and crime to survive! The occasional rounding up of sex workers in Kisumu Town, South Africa, has shown that a large percentage of the young females on the streets are orphaned children.[2]

Emma Guest describes this situation so well in her book, *Children of AIDS : Africa's Orphan Crisis*. "The growing phenomenon of child-headed households scraping for survival shows the determination of the remnants of families to stay together, living off the kindness of strangers and the scant attention of social workers. This forces them to engage in a variety of casual jobs to earn a living. They are usually exploited or taken advantage of, hence the loss of trust in the society that is supposed to protect

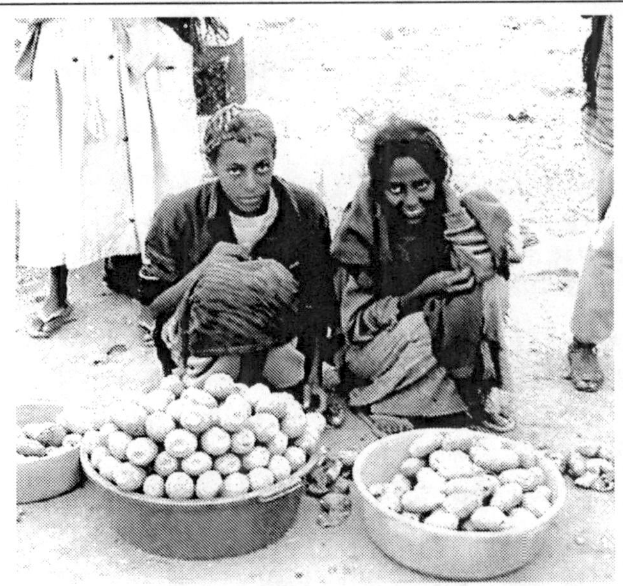

Pic. 4-1: Selling fruit is one way to survive

them. This compels them to grow up overnight to face adult responsibilities and the harsh realities of life: caring for younger siblings, with hardly enough to survive".[3]

Much less has been written about the way children manage the challenges that their lives present to them and how they themselves, by their actions, turn some of the challenges to good effect.[4] Many of these children are very industrious. In Pic. 4-1 are some girls selling fruits they have picked from bushes along the roadside.

And a young boy selling some eggs in Pic. 4-2. He came to the Sisters of St. Lucy at six years of age with his only other living relative, his 3-year-old brother. Sister started him on selling six eggs at a time. He now has his own house and a yard of chicks that support the two of them in good style.

Gavan O'Sullivan, in his doctoral thesis, says that even though children play a vital economic role, their own contribution is often played down as insignificant.[5] AIDS is responsible for pushing a significant percentage of children into the labor market.

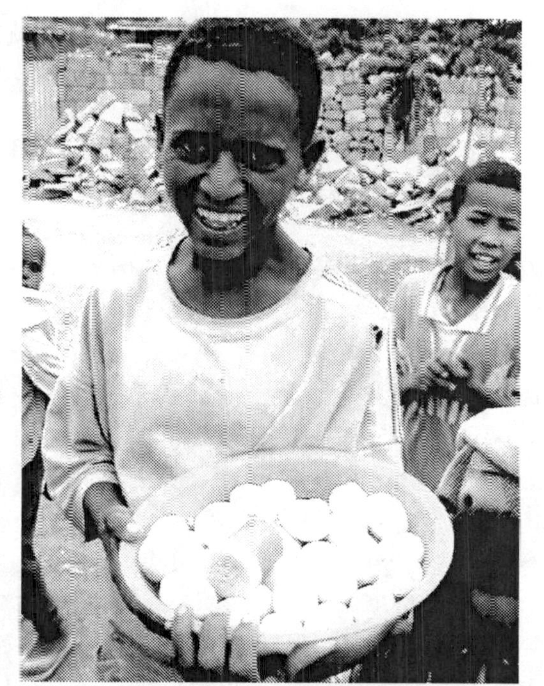

Pic. 4-2: Entrepreneur, since the age of 6, he provides for himself and three siblings

The kinds of help these children need includes:[6]

- Practical nutritional, health and financial or material assistance, including ensuring the security of tenure of the family in the house
- Developmental, emotional, spiritual and social support
- Ensuring that education, training and recreational needs are met, including lobbying for free education for households below a certain income
- Facilitating guardianship arrangements
- Training in agriculture, looking after animals.

Kenya's National Policy on Orphans and Vulnerable Children[7]

"Education is a fundamental right, and keeping children in school has been shown to reduce the risk of acquiring HIV infection as well as of early marriage, early sexual involvement, etc. Strategies in this area will include:

- Ensuring that OVC are enrolled in and complete basic education.
- Strengthening support programmes for OVC, including school feeding, health, bursaries, shelter, care and protection.
- Establishing non-formal education options, especially for working children.
- Extending the provision of bursaries for OVC to attend secondary schools even at constituency level, with due regard being given to gender.
- Providing text books and uniforms as a way of removing barriers to access to schooling for OVCs.
- Initiating flexible schooling options and reviewing school attendance requirements, like uniforms.
- Strengthening and supporting initiatives to achieve gender parity in education.
- Supporting HIV/AIDS mainstreaming into the school curriculum.
- Improving HIV/AIDS information access to OVC.
- Improving institutional capacity of existing schools in order to accommodate OVCs.
- Ensuring that early childhood development becomes a component of free education

The FOST study of CHH in Zimbabwe found that most children were able to complete their primary education but the older children at secondary level were more likely to be forced to drop out before they completed. There are several reasons for this. Firstly, primary education is much cheaper and it is also easier to get support for primary school fees. In addition, older siblings reported that having the younger children at school freed them to go to work.

Primary School fees ranged from Z$ 100 per term to a maximum of Z$ 300. Secondary school fees are normally more than 10 times the price of primary and there is much more pressure to wear school uniforms and purchase books and stationery.[8]

There is strong evidence from more qualitative sources that direct costs are one of the most important causes of non-attendance and early dropout from school. School costs are reported to be significant in this respect in China, Egypt, Ghana, Indonesia, Mexico, Pakistan and, for girls, in Bangladesh. In Malawi, from over 1,000 primary-school dropouts interviewed, half of the boys from rural areas and 44% of the boys from urban areas cited the lack of money for school expenses as the main reason for their having left school prematurely. This was also the most important factor for girls, although a smaller proportion of girls than boys—about one-third in both rural and urban areas indicated this.

Children often also indicate their "need to work" as the dominant reason for leaving school. If these two sets of causes are combined—i.e., costs and income—a majority of children are typically found to cite economic circumstances as the main reasons for their having left school. They accounted for 75% of the school dropouts interviewed in Zambia, 70% in Uganda and Ethiopia, 57% in Ghana, 45% in Malawi and 40% in Guinea[24]. In Tajikistan, in 2002, 68% of parents surveyed considered family poverty and the increased costs of education as the primary reason for girls' non-attendance.

Finally, separate evidence is available from a wide range of sources on the importance of household income as a determinant of school enrolments. In Senegal, the enrolment of children aged 6–14 from the poorest households is 52 percentage points lower than for those from the richest households. In Zambia there is a 36-percentage point gap. Here too there are gender differences: in Ethiopia, increasing a household's wealth index by one unit increases a boy's chances of attending school by 16%, whereas a girl's chances are increased by 41%. In Guinea, whereas the effect is insignificant for boys, girls' chances are increased by 9%. These results indicate that poverty in a family will have a more detrimental effect on the decision to enroll a girl in school than a boy.

For all these reasons, measures to reduce the direct costs of schooling are one of the most potent ways of increasing school enrolments—particularly for poorer households, and particularly for girls. There is ample experience, now, of the potentially huge numbers of children who may enroll in school when costs are sharply reduced.[9]

In the vast majority of cases, afflicted households do not "cope" in the sense of succeeding to preserve an acceptable livelihood, but rather they "struggle" and in fact commonly dissolve entirely.[10]

But this book is not about the children who are just coping. Coping, as defined by Barnett and Whiteside (2002), is escaping the challenges confronting them. Luzze shows that the children living in a child headed households can cope better than we think they can, particularly with the right amount of adult support. The problem is that children in child-headed households often lack adult support and supervision. He shows that there are 58 different coping mechanisms that the CHH employ to meet their activities of daily living.[11] But the CHH—these AIDS Orphans on the Rise—are not just coping or responding: they have a resilience way beyond their years.

The International Resilience Project defines resilience as a universal capacity that allows a person, group or community to prevent, minimize or overcome the damaging effects of adversity. Resilience may transform or make

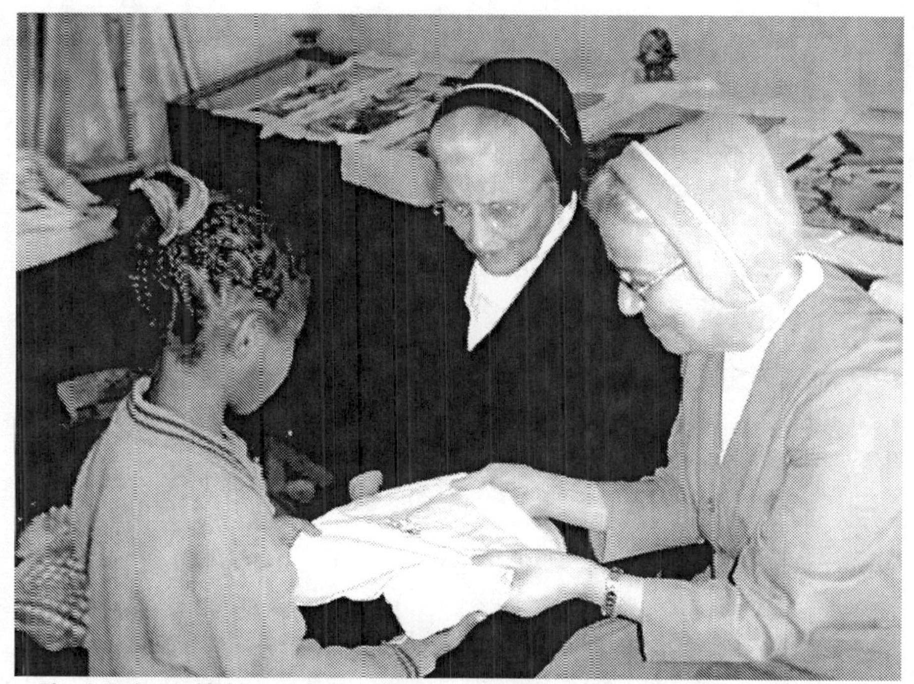

Pic. 4-3: Beautiful handwork brings in some money for this little girl and her family

stronger the lives of those who are resilient. The resilient behavior may be in response to adversity in the form of maintenance or normal development despite the adversity, or a promoter of growth beyond the present level of functioning. Further, resilience may be promoted not necessarily because of adversity, but, indeed, may be developed in anticipation of inevitable adversities.

Resilience does not develop in a vacuum; it is within a context. As children become older they appear to assume a larger role in the promotion of their own resilience, still in the context of their supports, their acquired skills, and their enhanced inner strengths. The challenge, then, is how to help the head of the CHH promote resilience to their siblings and become more resilient themselves.[12]

The resilient ones are going to make it in this world and be happy and productive citizens. But they need our help. There are many programs presently even if unknowingly reinforcing the resiliency of the CHH in their care. The program at St. Lucy School in Adigrat, Ethiopia, allows the young children to complete their elementary school education for free while also learning a trade. In Pic. 4-3, a young girl is showing the Sisters her handwork that will be sold. She will receive her earnings that will help raise her three younger siblings. St. Lucy School will continue to educate her and hundreds like her until she is old enough to live on her own with her younger brothers and sisters.

The UNICEF reports that most of the orphans are teenage girls. The announcement that girls and young women now account for 75 per cent of all Africans aged 15-24 living with HIV and AIDS, he said, "is unprecedented in the history of the pandemic and... perhaps the most ominous warning of what is yet to come."[13]

St. Lucy School provides for girls to receive their elementary school diploma and to receive a certificate in a skill that will help them to earn a living in an honorable manner. They will be able to support not only themselves but also provide for their younger siblings. The Sisters will help the students set up their own micro enterprise[14] or find a good job in the city. The Sisters have been doing this program for years with the *war widows* in Asmara, Eritrea and we have begun to replicate this program in Adigrat, Zalambessa, Goala, Sassi and soon at our newest school in the capital, Addis Ababa, Ethiopia.

What You Can Do To Help Now!

- Say a quick prayer for these children and all who are helping them.
- Bring clothes for children to a shelter where there are children—shoes, flip-flops and sneakers are very much needed.
- Get involved or start a training course for children; if there is something you do to make money they can learn from you.
- Send a sewing machine to a group that teaches young girls to sew.
- Send some hand tools to a group that teaches young boys different trades, like carpentry or mechanics.
- Start your own non-profit organization to help these CHH learn survival skills; go to http://www.GrantMeRich.com to learn how.
- Send a check or donate online to an organization that helps CHH with training the children.
- Send an email to all in your address book explaining the plight of these children and what they can do to help them.

5 What's Best for Them?

The number of AIDS orphans will nearly double to 25 million by 2010

Several things can happen to children when their parents die from HIV and AIDS-related causes. Firstly, they may be absorbed and assimilated into another existing family or household, usually that of a female relative. This is the most ideal because it often means that there is minimum disruption to the children's lives after the death of their parents. Unfortunately, however, widespread increasing poverty and economic hardships in our communities mean that this is happening less and less.[1]

Girls are often taken away by relatives and are more easily absorbed in other families than boys. This is particularly so because when old enough, most girls work in their new adopted homes as house helpers. Also upon growing up, girls get married and move away from the home. Hence, they are not permanent members of the home and do not pose long-term competition for family resources with caregivers' own children.[2]

As we have mentioned, grandmothers and even great grandmothers are taking on the responsibility of looking after orphans left by their children and grandchildren. Adoption or fostering of children of CHH who are not relatives is a possibility. It is common for parents in many sub-Saharan African countries to send their children to be raised away from home, either by relatives or by non-relatives. They may do this because they are unable to take care of the children themselves, to save money, or to

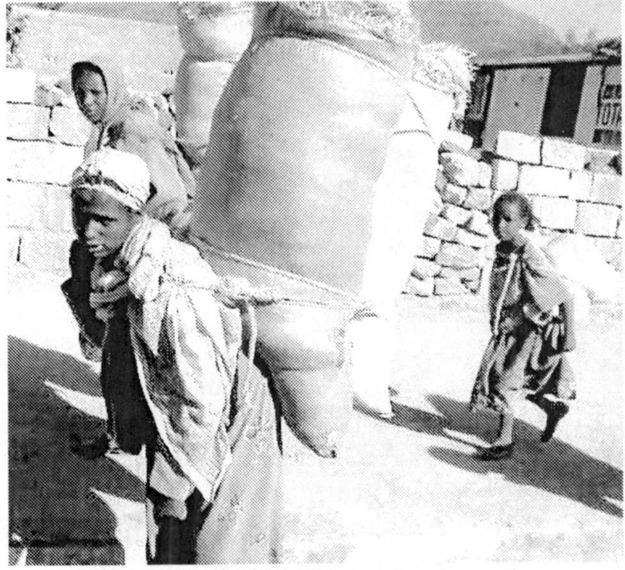

Pic. 5-1: Some kids work harder than others

provide their children with better economic opportunities. The foster family also gains from this arrangement since it can acquire child workers, particularly for domestic service. In some countries, a high proportion of children, 20 per cent or more, may not be living with their parents.[3]

The deeply rooted tradition of child fostering within the extended family may be one of the main reasons for the slow development of adoption in much of Africa. In some contexts, taboos and cultural beliefs also may discourage people from taking unrelated children into their home. In Zimbabwe, the fear of invoking *ngozi* (the avenging spirit) is strong. In South Africa, obstacles such as tribal allegiances and animism mitigate against adoption. Some anecdotal evidence suggests that in specific contexts, fostering and adoption by unrelated families have increased without any external support. For example, after the 1994 genocide in Rwanda, many families fostered unrelated children. The fostering was perceived to be a moral imperative because so many children were orphaned.[4]

Throughout sub-Saharan Africa, there have been traditional systems in place to take care of children who lose their parents for various reasons. But the onslaught of HIV slowly but surely erodes this good traditional practice by simply overloading its caring capacity by the sheer number of orphaned children needing support and care. HIV also undermines the caring capacity of families and communities by deepening poverty due to loss of labor and the high cost of medical treatment and funerals.[5]

> The second initiative, our *Staff "Adopt" an Orphan Programme,* has been enthusiastically received with 313 orphans being financially supported through monthly contributions from 189 of our staff members.
>
> ...from part of *Old Mutual's* citizenship transformation programme[6]

Adoption from a Distance

Many organizations have been offering the possibility of adopting a distant child for years. Note in the box, even *Old Mutual* has such a program! A person sends so much money per month and receives several reports and pictures each year from the child they have been supporting. The advantages of this system are that they keep the child in its own environment and near their brothers and sisters and any relatives that might still be living. Reputable organizations, like Angel Covers, use the money wisely and provide food, medicine and education for the children. It is wise to investigate the group you are aiding. How much of your money actually gets to the child? Will the child really receive the money or is it put into a pot where the child will get some help but not more than the others?

Is the picture you are receiving actually the child receiving your gift, or have they sent this same picture to hundreds of others? Often it is better to give a monthly sum to an organization designated for food, clothing, education—whatever you wish for the children. The money you send for one child even if only ten dollars could buy bread for 400 children. Money goes a long way in these very poor countries. Investigate well.

International Adoption

Melissa Fay Greene's article in the *New York Times Magazine* depicts very clearly the real situation and the good being done for Ethiopian orphans at Layla House.

"Layla House, a shady compound with a paved common area, a baby house, dormitories for boys and for girls, a schoolroom and a kitchen and dining hall, is run by Adoption Advocates International, based in Port Angeles, Wash. A.F.A.A. House, on the outskirts of town, almost buried in flower gardens, is run by Americans for African Adoptions, based in Indianapolis and directed by Cheryl Carter-Shotts. These two are the only American agencies permitted by the Ethiopian government to arrange for adoption of healthy Ethiopian orphans to America. More than 100 children joined new families in the U.S. in 2001.

At least a dozen other adoption agencies based in Addis Ababa represent Australia, Canada and seven nations of Western Europe and Scandinavia. It is the first recourse of everyone ethically involved with inter-country adoption to place orphans with relatives, with friends or with families within their home countries; no one imagines or pretends that adoption is a solution to a generation of children orphaned by disease. It is one very small and modest option, a case of families in industrialized nations throwing lifelines to individual children even as their governments fail to commit the money to turn back the epidemic."[7]

Global Alliance for Africa, operating in Chicago since 1996, has provided care for more than 1,000 AIDS orphans in Kenya and Tanzania by providing safe environments in extended family or foster care homes.

In addition to caretaker family placement, the Global Alliance program, in conjunction with local African non-governmental partners, provides school fees, school uniforms, health care, and psychosocial support monitored

Angel Covers offers several sponsorship programs as a part of their mission to help children around the world. As a sponsor you can make a direct impact on in a child's life. Through your sponsorship, a child could attend school for the first time, have enough food to eat, and will know that someone cares about their future. Each of our sponsorship programs is slightly different, allowing you to choose the one that best suits your abilities. You may choose to sponsor a child who is not able to receive letters and packages, or you may want the ability to write, send gifts, and maybe visit your child someday. Find the sponsorship program that meets your desires to get involved and change the life of a child today![8]

Visit this site to learn more about International adoptions:
http://www.adoptionadvocates.org/AAI/Home.htm

closely by local staff members. The program also arranges for caretaker families to participate in economic development initiatives that help support the child, according to Global Alliance Executive Director Tom Derdak.[9]

In Bangalore, India, there is finally some hope for children rendered destitute by HIV in their parents but who have tested negative for the virus. Adoption agencies and the Voluntary Coordinating Agency, which facilitates in-country adoption, have come forward to help them. These children will now be placed in a few adoption agencies in Bangalore.[10]

Officials at times falsely claim that there are enough families within their own country to adopt or take care of the orphans, according to a recent posting from Africa's Angels: "During my recent visit, I found that there were some people in positions of significance who strongly felt there were enough adoptive families within South Africa for all of South Africa's orphans. Although I wish this were true, I spent nearly two weeks visiting packed orphanages, children's homes and other children's centers, and I found that this is simply not the case."

I believe much of the resistance to international adoption is out of concern that children being adopted from South Africa will lose their culture when placed outside their native country. While I can appreciate the desire to maintain a child's culture, I still believe that when a loving adoptive home is not available for an orphan within their own country, it is in the best interest of the child to be placed with any available loving adoptive home, even if that family does not reside in South Africa. It is important that families who adopt internationally, or trans-racially, actively take steps to teach their child about their country and culture of birth. There is no reason this cannot be done while the child is safe with a loving family they can call their own.[11]

Institutional - Residential Care

The hardships faced by AIDS orphans have been documented for more than a decade, and African governments are trying to develop and implement solutions. Some have created new laws and policies to protect children and to help women and children defend their inheritance and rights to property, and have provided child advocates to help children redress exploitation. While governments also try to offer adoption and fostering stipends, public welfare assistance, and access to education and health services for poor children and families perhaps only 2% of needy families have access to such government safety nets.

Governments still generally rely on communities and volunteers to provide the bulk of social services for AIDS orphans and families. Orphanages, hospices, and other institutions in a developing country have the estimated capacity to take perhaps 5% of AIDS and non-AIDS orphans in institutional care.[12]

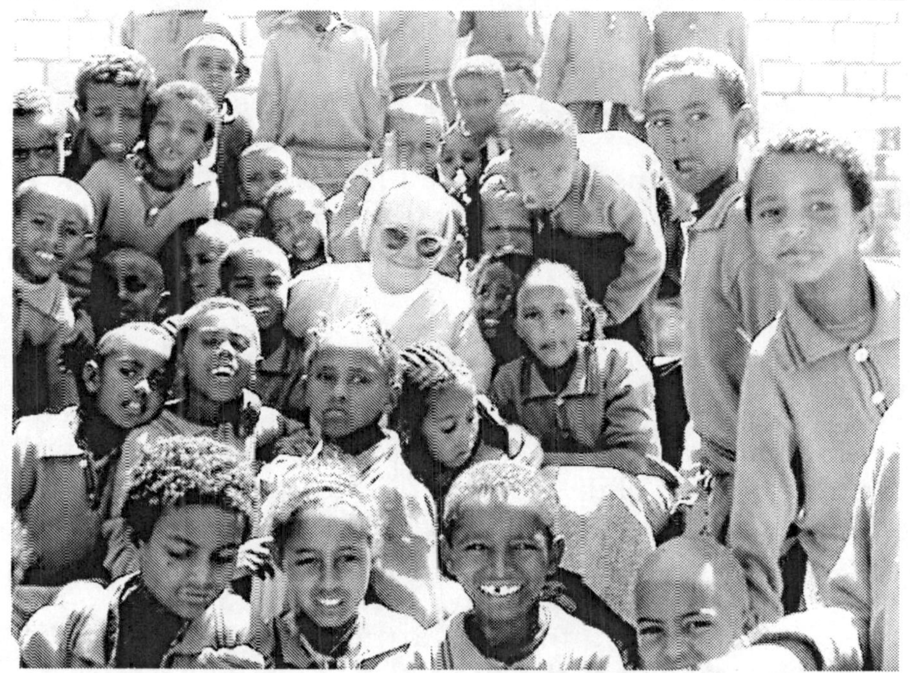

Pic. 5-2: Sr. Antonia enjoying the children she has been helping for 40 years

"Only in America!" -- From *Johns Hopkins Magazine*

In dismantling the orphanage system, Progressive reformers laid the groundwork for modern welfare--the same welfare system that some reformers today want to fix (you guessed it!) by bringing back the orphanage. Crenson's research has resulted in a forthcoming book, The Invisible Orphanage: A Pre-history of the American Welfare System. In that book he examines how the turn-of-the-century Progressive Movement championed child-care reforms that led to the dismantling of the orphanage system. He says, "People are going to give me an argument about this, but I believe that in the process of dismantling the orphanages, what society did, albeit indirectly, was activate the institutional apparatus for welfare." [13]

In Africa, institutional care for orphans is quite limited; only 1–3% of orphans are cared for in institutional settings. With the sharp increase in orphans in Africa and the process of deinstitutionalization, new and innovative forms of institutional or semi-institutional care have emerged, such as children's homes and children's villages. But these forms vary widely in size, management, and effectiveness.[14]

Learn from History

Timothy Hacsi's *Second Home Orphan Asylums and Poor Families in America* is a well researched and well written account of the rise and decline of orphan asylums in America. It is a heartfelt and subtle argument about the best ways in which a society can care for its dependent children. As orphan asylums ceased to exist in the late twentieth century, interest in them dwindled as well. Yet, from the Civil War to the Great Depression, America's dependent children—children whose families were unable to care for them—received more aid from orphan asylums than through any other means. The asylums spread widely and endured because different groups—churches, ethnic communities, charitable organizations, fraternal societies, and local and state governments—could adapt them to their own purposes.[15]

> A survey by Richard McKenzie, a University of California at Irvine business professor who grew up in an orphanage in North Carolina, polled hundreds of orphanage alumni and found them to be happier, healthier and wealthier than the average American.[16]

There is a critical need to develop sustainable community based models that address the scale of the problem and provide quality and comprehensive care. Save the Children UK and local governments are developing a program of Orphans and other Vulnerable Children (OVC) care in one poor municipality in South Africa. They have been able to establish and train child care forums (CCFs) in all of the municipality's 34 wards in 9 months. The CCFs are community groups whose role is to identify vulnerable children, mobilize community support for the children and link them to services and resources.[17]

The Kgaitsadi Society in Gabarone is an example of a community organization set up to care for and educate AIDS orphans. Started in 2002, it assists with their basic needs and provides basic and primary school level education through a flexible school program. It also provides support for children caring for family members and for those who are working. Other examples of community organizations are the Maun Counseling Centre, and the House of Hope in Palapye, both of which provide day care support for orphans.

Save the Children in Malawi mobilizes and helps more than 200 village committees that care for about 23,000 orphans and others in AIDS-stricken areas; the program is serving as a model for similar efforts in Ethiopia, Mali, and Mozambique.[18]

Many shy away from increasing the number of orphanages or other forms of institutional care because it is economically impossible, given the degree of national debt and poverty that most African governments already face. Caring for a child in an Ethiopian orphanage costs between $300-500 per year—more than three times the nation's average per capita income.

Community-based support projects for orphans are becoming common. A Ugandan project launched by Janet Museveni, wife of President Yoweri Museveni in 1986, assists orphans in resettlement camps and returns them to their extended families. Museveni's organization also helps fund education and training for the children and provides credit to caretakers to start small businesses and trading activities.[19]

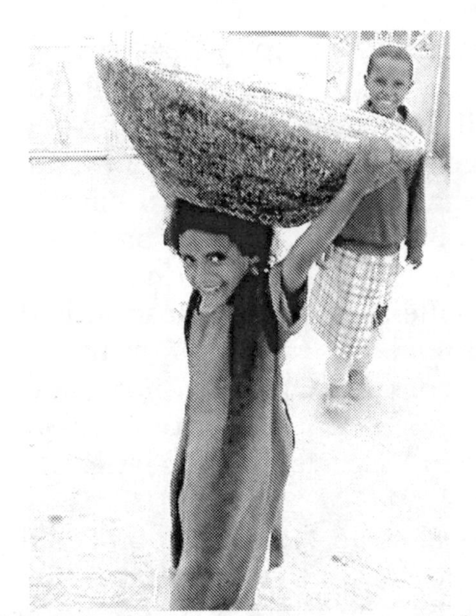

Pic. 5-3: Selling grain is one way to support a family

Although many experts[20] agree that caring for orphans within the community is the better and cheaper option, there are now an ever-increasing number of orphanages, homes, transit homes and children's villages. These are the formal institutions that take in children orphaned by AIDS; some of them actually deliberately target children who are not only affected by AIDS with the death of their parents, but those orphans who are themselves infected with HIV, even those who have AIDS. These institutions range from houses in the townships and suburbs looking after several children, to elaborate "villages" with several houses, schools, playground and clinics. They are run by individuals, families, NGOs, churches, missions, and other charities

The Red Cross is not in favor of institutional care such as orphanages, except as a last resort or a temporary measure.[21] The best interests of the child must be the primary consideration when deciding where the child will live after the parent dies.

Institutionalized care for the majority of orphans and other affected children is not an appropriate option. Resources are more effectively used in strengthening the abilities of families and communities to care for orphaned and affected children in their midst. Where institutional care is offered, programs must be developed to integrate children back into their communities at the earliest opportunity.[22] Furthermore, institutional care is not a socially acceptable solution in the African culture. Many African countries depend on a subsistence economy, and children sent from their village may lose rights to their parents' land. In addition, an institutionalized orphan would be removed from the companionship of any remaining siblings and their community. In Zimbabwe, where AIDS has orphaned 7% of all children under the age of 15, the National Policy advocates that orphans be cared for by the community whenever possible and only placed in institutions as a last resort. Most surrounding eastern and southern African countries have also taken a stance against building more orphanages because it drains resources needed to support family and community-based programs.[23]

And yet, it was found that Malawian orphans placed in orphanages have an advantage over those placed in foster homes along the dimensions of lodging, health care, food quantity and variety, clothing and school supplies. Additionally, children in orphanages have more autonomy, and have a broader concept of their future potential. Orphanage residents view their caregivers as compassionate and loving. Finally, it was found that orphanages are more efficient in providing care and at exchanging information with other organizations. They are also easier to replicate for use in other areas than are community-based programs.[24]

Kalanidhi Subbarao and Diane Coury, in *Reaching Out to Africa's Orphans: A Framework for Public Action*[25] present a study aimed at addressing the needs of young children affected by loss of one or both parents as a consequence of HIV/AIDS and conflicts. In doing so, it makes a substantial contribution to our understanding of the many risks and vulnerabilities faced by orphans and the ameliorating role played by governments and donors.

Kwami Saka believes that residential care, whether statutory or non-statutory, is the least preferred care arrangement for AIDS orphans and vulnerable children as against placements of orphans with family members.[26] Almost all sub-Saharan African governments, international NGOs, development local policy makers and practitioners have agreed to the description and position that residential care is "the last resort."

However, not only has there been no empirical basis for this above assertion, but also, other care options have failed to make any significant improvements in the lives of AIDS orphans and other vulnerable children. Also, we now know that formal placement of orphans with family members more often than not does fail, and when it does, its impact on the orphan is devastating because the orphan completely loses trust in any body or organization.

Similarly, both non-statutory and formal residential homes also have their problems. Yet, given the fact that the traditional care systems are struggling to cope with chronic poverty added to the orphan crisis, they can no longer be relied upon to efficiently and effectively take care of orphans and vulnerable children.

Each care option has the potential to meet the needs, interests and rights of orphans and other vulnerable children. We must deal with each case on its own terms, taking into consideration contextual and structural factors which may promote or hinder care and service delivery to AIDS orphans and other vulnerable children.

Child Headed Households Living by Themselves

We have been discussing placing AIDS orphans in some type of care, whether foster or institutional. But this book has been written for the CHH who are out there living and *making it* on their own. They don't have AIDS, but they have a love of life and a deep love for their siblings. Give these CHH a chance to stay together as a family and make it on their own! An outrageous idea? Not if there could be some adult supervision in the area that they can go to when they need help, and if these supervisors check in on them daily to see that they have all that they need.

At this time, there are too many CHH out there *making it* to view them as helpless. And with the latest study compiled by UN children's agency UNICEF and the US development agency USAID, based on data from 88 countries in Africa, Asia, Latin America and the Caribbean that claims the number of AIDS orphans will nearly double to 25 million by 2010, we must examine the strategies that the children are using not just to cope but to move on to a great life ahead of them so that others can learn from them. The silent power many children wield is that of resilience and endurance in coping with very challenging circumstances. It is possible with appropriate support from NGOs and other community support systems for orphans to be nurtured in CHH.[27]

The CHH have the advantage that children are not separated from their brothers and sisters to live with different relatives. Research in Zambia found the separation of siblings to be a significant factor in psychosocial distress among orphans. Remaining in their parents' house is also a way for children to retain possession of the land, support themselves and maintain a sense of continuity in their lives. In many cases, these children will continue to receive the support and guidance of the community.[28]-

Many advocate to keep the siblings together no matter what the circumstances, yet there are times when it is not possible or not even safe for the siblings to remain together. Becky Malecki from Colorado State University, once adamant about keeping displaced siblings together, gives some very strong reasons why some siblings should not stay together.

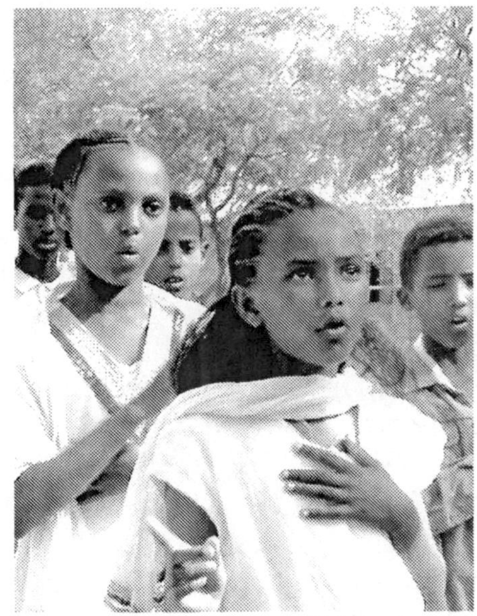

Pic. 5-4: Teenage girls learn many things, even how to sing!

"In the case of a relatively normal, well-functioning sibling group, they should be kept together—e.g., when a parent has died from AIDS or some other illness, and the children do trust adults, then I would fully support it. However, in scenarios involving abuse and neglect, with resulting attachment disorder, I think keeping siblings together is often counterproductive to helping the children to heal. First work on their healing. Keep them in contact with one another. When they are healed, then is the time to establish meaningful relationships. In other words, contrary to my initial beliefs, I now know that it's often absolutely necessary to separate young siblings! Children need to bond to a loving adult in order to ever be able to deal with issues of trust, authority or real intimacy. A bond with an unhealthy sibling often stands in the way of the parent-child bond. It can be used as a crutch—I don't need you, I've got my brother in much the same way gang members rely on each other for a sense of belonging and security."

The Religious Teachers Filippini, working with the CHH of Adigrat, recognized that the very young CHH should be in a hostel or group home where they can still live together as a family within the confines of a protected setting. These young CHH are provided an education and the older children are given technical skills so they are able to make a living once they leave the Sisters. The Sisters do all they can to protect their inheritance, most especially any land that might be rightfully theirs. The children are encouraged and given the opportunity to visit any remaining relatives. These children are assured of housing until they have a secure position in the work force and are ready to go on their own.

As the research indicates, it is inevitable the number of CHH will increase tremendously over the next few years, but with proper guidance, schooling and love these children can grow to be caring adults and have the ability to turn Africa into a productive continent.

Human Rights Instruments

The African Charter is aimed at the advancement of children's rights and the protection of their welfare. The idea to develop an African Charter on the rights of the child emanated from a conference organized by ANPPCAN and supported by UNICEF on Children in Situations of Armed Conflict in Africa in 1987. The Charter entered into force 12 years later Nov. 29, 1999, in time to benefit the millions of orphans from AIDS. If this Charter is adhered to, many children will be able to thrive and to one day bring Africa to its proper place in the world.

> Article 7 of the African Charter: Every child who is capable of communicating his or her own views shall be assured the rights to express his opinions freely in all matters and to disseminate his opinions subject to such restrictions as are prescribed by laws.[29]

Ironically, children had no part in the drafting of the African Charter, nor are they being consulted on how to implement the articles, yet reading Article 7 one sees clearly that the document recognizes the children's capabilities. It is important to make children part of the solution in tackling the AIDS pandemic; they are generally left out of making important decisions. Children and young people are virtually invisible in terms of public policy and of voices expressed on the national stage. Research on risk and resilience among children in developed countries has shown that a significant proportion of children exposed to highly stressful situations remain quite resilient even in the long term.[30] Children's experiences of adversity are mediated by a host of internal and external factors that are inseparable from the social, political, and economic contexts in which children live.

Serious doubt is being cast on the relevance of many traditional prescriptions for protecting children, especially interventions imposed from outside the child's social and cultural context.

The idea that children might take an active part in decision-making is still very novel; others may fear the consequences. Frederick Luzze is convinced that as long as the orphan crisis continues, and more and more CHHs continue to emerge, the acceptance of the CHH as an alternative mode of orphan care is inevitable for the time being. It is possible with appropriate support from NGOs and other community support systems for orphans to be nurtured in CHHs.

Children need to be acknowledged as contributing citizens of the Africa of today. They cannot just be targets of interventions designed by adults far away from the everyday reality which confronts these children.

Children on the Brink (2004) presents a simple strategic framework for action that emphasizes the importance of strengthening the capacity of children to meet their own needs as part of facilitating primary responses within a comprehensive HIV/AIDS strategy.[31]

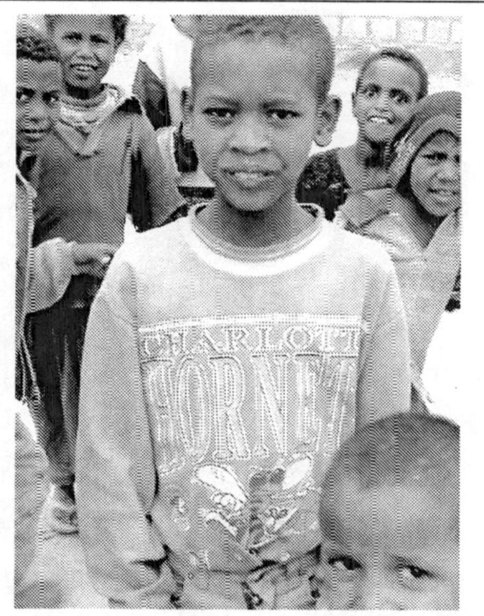

Pic. 5-5: Boys taking the role of men

So many countries in Africa are still a long way from making the African Charter on the Rights and Welfare of the Child (ACRWC) into reality. Is it political will, or economics? The numbers of health and economic problems that these African nations are dealing with are overwhelming their capability to deal with the orphan issue. Those nations where all the children are enjoying basic good health, and are receiving an education, can help Africa in so many ways, if there is the will. Tsunamis, hurricanes, tornadoes draw our attention, as many of our own families are suffering. But the orphan children are still there and need help. It is so very hard to keep them upfront in our minds. Some of us know someone with AIDS and we see them getting treatment, so the idea of thousands of parents dying from the disease is so foreign, the orphans are only a picture or perhaps an infomercial on a remote cable channel. Please don't delay. Do what you can to help these children now!

> The challenge of dealing with so many orphans requires dedication to ensure that what we articulate in terms of policy provides quality interventions. We need to be very careful, willing to take time, and not be too quick to decide, because a wrong policy that affects children is worse than no policy at all. Anything that affects our children affects our future. If it is bad, so will our future be. If it is good, so will our future be.
>
> Janet Museveni, First lady of Uganda[32]

What You Can Do To Help Now!

- Say a quick prayer for these children and all who are helping them.
- Call someone who has adopted a child and ask if they need any help.
- Go online and see how many adoption sites there are specific for CHH; often just clicking on a group's site helps them to raise money.
- Write to adoption agencies who do not help CHH and encourage them to do so.
- Look into adoption procedures for yourself: contact the Missionaries of Charity in Addis Ababa, Ethiopia.
- Look into adopting from a distance.
- Start your own non-for profit organization to help the CHH children get adopted as a family help to keep them together. Learn how at www.GrantMeRich.com.
- Contact sites where they house CHH to ask them what you might do to help.
- Send toys, soccer balls, etc. to group homes or hostels that help CHH.

- Send school supplies—pencils, crayon, chalk—to organizations that house CHH.
- Collect from friends or relatives or contact a local elementary school and ask if you might have a clothes drive for these children; often local Women's Clubs will donate money for shipping.
- Send a check or donate online to an organization that helps CHH; be sure to indicate you want it to go only for the housing or adoption of a CHH.
- Send an email or this book to everyone in your address book explaining the plight of these children.

6 What Will You Do?

If you have read this far, then you are serious about learning about the orphans from AIDS. Are you serious about helping them?

> **If I look at the masses, I will never act.**
> **If I look at the one, I will.**
>
> **Mother Teresa**

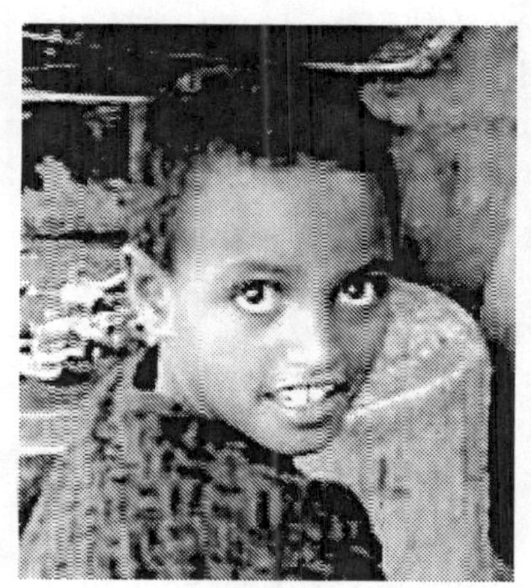

Pic. 6-1

Well, here is one you can help! She is the face of millions orphans, not just from Africa but in a growing number of countries throughout this world.

The HIV epidemic shows no sign of disappearing. The world needs a strong wakeup call before the present orphans and the millions more to come grow up without not just the proper food, water, healthcare, clothes and basic education, but without love, a sense of belonging, acceptance or any core values. Most of all they need a "formation of the heart."[1] There is not one solution to these problems. There are many solutions! Governments are not the ones to solve this problem. The governments can provide the monetary and policy actions, but the actual caring interventions for the children will need to be adapted to the culture and context for each child. This unprecedented crisis will require an extraordinary community response including NGOs, religious groups and private initiatives. They must be given the support they need to help these children.

To live is to choose. But to choose well, these children must know who they are and what they stand for, where do they want to go in life, and why do they want to get there.[2] The challenge is not to just avoid a catastrophe but to ensure that these children be given the capability to make the best of their lives here on earth.

"If I give away all I have, and if I deliver my body to be burned, but do not have love, I gain nothing" (I Corinthians 13). Not only will you gain nothing, but the children know when people are just throwing money at them. They need love more than all of your money. But how, you ask, can I give them love 1000 miles or more away? Perhaps the words of Pope Benedict XVI, found in his latest encyclical *Deus Caritas Est,* will help you understand what you should do for these children.

> "Practical activity will always be insufficient, unless it visibly expresses a love for man, a love nourished by an encounter with Christ. My deep personal sharing in the needs and sufferings of others becomes a sharing of my very self with them…
>
> "I must give to others not only something that is my own, but my very self I must be present personally in my gift."[3]

At the end of each of the previous chapters you were asked to pray for these children. Some are wondering, "What good will that do?" And when we are asked to make a sacrifice, like eat your peas for the starving children of Africa, do these acts of piety mean anything?

Pope Benedict explains that people who pray are not wasting time, even though the situation appears desperate and seems to call for action alone. Piety does not undermine the struggle against the poverty of our neighbors, however extreme. In the example of Blessed Teresa of Calcutta, we have a clear illustration of the fact that time devoted to God in prayer not only does not detract from effective and loving service to our neighbor but is in fact the inexhaustible source of that service.

We contribute to a better world only by personally doing good now, with full commitment and wherever we have the opportunity, independently of partisan strategies and programs. The Christian's program like the program of the Good Samaritan, is "a heart which sees." This heart sees where love is needed and acts accordingly.

Following the example given in the parable of the Good Samaritan, Christian charity is first of all the simple response to immediate needs and specific situations: feeding the hungry, clothing the naked, caring for and healing the sick, visiting those in prison, etc. There will never be a situation where the charity of each individual Christian is unnecessary, because in addition to justice man needs, and will always need, love.

These children need love more than anything else, and governments are not equipped to provide love. Love can come only from those of us who care.

Whoever wants to eliminate love is preparing to eliminate man as such. There will always be suffering that cries out for consolation and help. There will always be loneliness. There will always be situations of material need where help in the form of concrete love of neighbor is indispensable. The State that would provide everything, absorbing everything into itself, would ultimately become a mere bureaucracy incapable of guaranteeing the very thing which the suffering person—every person—needs: namely, loving personal concern. We do not need a State that regulates and controls everything, but a State which, in accordance with the principle of subsidiarity, generously acknowledges and supports initiatives arising from the different social forces and combines spontaneity with closeness to those in need.

The Church is one of those living forces: she is alive with the love enkindled by the Spirit of Christ. This love does not simply offer people material help, but refreshment and care for their souls, something which often is even more necessary than material support. In the end, the claim that just social structures would make works of charity superfluous masks a materialist conception of man: the mistaken notion that man can live "by bread alone" (Mt 4:4; cf. Dt 8:3)—a conviction that demeans man and ultimately disregards all that is specifically human.

Prayer for the Child Headed Households

Mary Immaculate Virgin, Woman of pain and hope, be benevolent to the children who suffer and obtain for them fullness of life. Turn your maternal gaze especially to those children who are in extreme need. Look kindly and help the grandparents who are without sufficient resources to support their grandchildren who have become orphans. Look at the siblings living together huddled alone never to feel a mother's touch. Clasp all of them to your maternal heart, and let them feel a mother's love. Most Holy Virgin, pray for us.

And in closing, the words of our beloved Pope John Paul II, a great example to all of us as he not only prayed for these children, but provided for their material needs by setting up special agencies within the Vatican to help them. He also traveled to 104 nations to visit them personally.

> "Children's faces should always be happy and trusting, but at times they are full of sadness and fear; how much have these children already seen and suffered in the course of their short lives. Let us give children a future of peace. This is the confident appeal which I make to men and women of good will, and I invite everyone to help children to grow up in an environment of authentic peace. This is their right, and it is our duty".[4]

References

How the Book Began

1. From a book review of *Children of AIDS: Africa's orphan crisis* by Emma Guest.
   http://www.iss.co.za/pubs/ASR/11No2/BookRev.html

Introduction

1. Youth and HIV/AIDS Facts
   http://www.unfpa.org/swp/2005/presskit/factsheets/facts_youth.htm
2. Guest, Emma, September 5, 2003 *Children of AIDS: Africa's Orphan Crisis, 2nd Ed.* Pluto Press.
3. Help Kenya's Orphans
   http://www.changethroughchildren.org/images/os/download/OSPposter.pdf
4. UNICEF Mother to Child Transmission
   http://www.unicef.org/publications/files/pub_factsheet_mtct_en.pdf
5. Children on the Brink 2004: A joint report of new orphan estimates and a framework for action
   http://www.unicef.org/publications/index_22212.html
6. Zambia and HIV/AIDS
   http://www.synergyAIDS.com/documents/554_Zambia.pdf
7. Goedgedacht Forum for Social Reflection. Summary notes from a debate held on 24 November 2001: "The emerging crisis of orphans and vulnerable children: strategic responses for faith-based community networks"
   http://www.goedgedacht.org.za/debates/011124.html

Chapter 1

1. Help Kenya's Orphans
   http://www.neasc.org/neasc/aed_orphan_support.htm
2. Africa's Orphaned Generations
   http://www.unicef.org/publications/files/africas_orphans.pdf

3. Social networks help Tanzanian children and caregivers cope with HIV/AIDS
http://www.crin.org/resources/infodetail.asp?id=7232
4. *Black Death: AIDS in Africa.* Susan Hunter 2003
http://www.amazon.com/dp/1403962448/
5. West and Central Africa Regional Workshop on Orphans and other Vulnerable Children Yamoussoukro, Côte d'Ivoire, 8-12 April 2002.
http://www.fhi.org/NR/rdonlyres/eemv5jig57m3hanpeu76kd6hzr2mjcn5mxxzxstvl3kku45ta5rn73pnjc4pp5slpk2cnpdh3tdcgn/FinalreportOVCworkshopApril02.pdf
6. Africa's Orphaned Generations
http://www.unicef.org/publications/files/africas_orphans.pdf
7. *HIV/AIDS: Does Uganda Really Show The Way Forward?* Doreen Kibuka-Musoke
http://www.open2.net/makingadifference/AIDS.htm
8. AIDS orphans - the facts.
http://www.avert.org/AIDSorphans.htm
9. From single parents to child-headed households: the case of children orphaned by AIDS in Kisumu and Siaya districts in Kenya. http://www.eldis.ids.ac.uk/static/DOC6292.htm
10. *Where AIDS orphans see prostitution as a way out for a living.* Mary Ombara
http://www.nationaudio.com/News/DailyNation/05072002/News/Spotlight4.html
11. What is child poverty?
http://www.savethechildren.org.uk/makechildpovertyhistory/
12. *Too little, too late? Provisioning for child-headed households"* Julia Sloth-Nielsen
http://www.communitylawcentre.org.za/ser/esr2002/2002july_child.php
13. Learn how world vision is helping the orphans
http://www.worldvision.org/
14. *Black Death: AIDS in Africa* Susan Hunter 2003.
http://www.amazon.com/gp/product/1403962448/104-3603845-1286323?v=glance&n=283155

15. *Youth Civic Engagement: Promise and Peril.* Scot Evans and Isaac Prilleltensky. To appear in M. Ungar (Ed.), *Pathways to resilience: A handbook of theory, methods, and interventions.* Sage. http://people.vanderbilt.edu/~isaac.prilleltensky/civic.htm

Chapter 2

1. Street children - What are street children? http://www.mexico-child-link.org/street-children-definition-statistics.htm
2. Levine, C. 1995. Today's challenges, tomorrow's dilemmas. In *Forgotten Children of the AIDS Epidemic*, ed. S.Geballe, J. Gruendel and W. Andiman. New Haven: Yale University Press.
3. Foster G., C. Makufa, R. Drew, and E. Kralovec. 1997a. Factors Leading to the Establishment of Child-Headed Households: The Case of Zimbabwe. *Health Transition Review* supplement 2,7: 155–168. http://htc.anu.edu.au/pdfs/Foster1.pdf
4. Women's Day/Health-Zimbabwe: Grandmothers Care for AIDS Orphans. http://www.accessmylibrary.com/comsite5/bin/pdinventory.pl?pdlanding=1&referid=2930&purchase_type=ITM&item_id=0286-6953917&word=WOMENS_DAY_HEALTH
5. From Single Parents to Child-Headed Households: The case of Children Orphaned by AIDS in Kisumu and Siaya Districts. http://www.undp.org/hiv/publications/study/english/sp7e.htm
6. Saoke, P., R. Mutemi and C. Blair 1996. Another Song Begins: Children Orphaned by AIDS. Pp. 45-64 in *AIDS in Kenya: Socio-economic Impact and Policy Implications*, ed. S. Forsythe and B. Rau. Arlington: Family Health International/AIDSCAP.
7. Introduction to AIDS in Zambia. http://www.avert.org/AIDS-zambia.htm
8. Durban Street Kids Project http://www.hopehiv.org/page/120/durban-street-kids-project.html
9. Africa's Orphaned Generations http://www.unicef.org/publications/files/africas_orphans.pdf

10. Researching the Experiences of HIV-AIDS orphans in Jozini KwaZulu-Natal http://66.249.93.104/search?q=cache:qjrnX0_jb7UJ:www.kznAID-Slink.kabissa.org/josini.doc+%22Their+educators,+during+my+school+visits,+confirmed+their+%22&hl=en&ct=clnk&cd=1
11. Brigitte Zimmerman http://www.stanford.edu/dept/publicpolicy/programs/Honors_Theses/Theses_2005/Zimmerman.pdf
12. Young AIDS migrants in Southern Africa: policy implications for empowering children. Young L, Ansell N. AIDS Care. 2003 Jun;15(3):337-45.
13. Foster G., C. Makufa, R. Drew, and E. Kralovec. 1997a. Factors Leading to the Establishment of Child-Headed Households: The Case of Zimbabwe. *Health Transition Review* supplement 2,7: 155–168. http://htc.anu.edu.au/pdfs/Foster1.pdf
14. Orphans & vulnerable children http://www.savethechildren.org.uk/scuk/jsp/whatwedo/subtheme.jsp?section=hivAIDS&subsection=orphansvulnerablechildren
15. AIDS Orphans http://www.bodyandmind.co.za/healthweb/AIDS_Orphans.html
16. SOS Children's Villages http://www.sos-childrensvillages.org/cgi-bin/sos/jsp/retrieve.do?lang=en&site=ZZ&nav=2.1
17. Orphans and other Children affected by HIV/AIDS http://www.unicef.org/publications/pub_factsheet_orphan_en.pdf
18. AIDS and Orphans: A Tragedy Unfolding http://www.unAIDS.org/bangkok2004/GAR2004_html/GAR2004_05_en.htm
19. Care for Orphans, Children Affected by HIV/AIDS, and Other Vulnerable Children http://www.fhi.org/en/HIVAIDS/pub/fact/carorphans.htm
20. World Vision is Helping the AIDS orphans http://www.worldvision.org/

21. Special Report of the Commission on Human Rights on Adequate Housing as a Component of the Right to an Adequate Standard of Living, and on the Right to Non-discrimination in this Context
http://www.ohchr.org/english/issues/housing/index.htm

22. Special Session Combating HIV/AIDS
http://www.unicef.org/specialsession

23. Habitat for Humanity, Comic Relief strive to help AIDS orphans
http://www.habitat.org/newsroom/2004archive/insitedoc006490.aspx

24. *Too little, too late? Provisioning for child-headed households* . Julia Sloth-Nielsen
http://www.communitylawcentre.org.za/ser/esr2002/2002july_child.php

25. Empowering AIDS orphans and Street Children
http://www.allforyouth.org/

26. O'Sullivan, Gavan *Starting from Strengths. Social Exclusion, Rights Based Approach and Children in Charge of Families Affected by HIV/AIDS in Uganda.* Dissertation submitted to: London School of Economics and Political Science University of London. September, 2003.

27. National Policy on Kenyan Orphans and Vulnerable Children
http://www.reliefweb.int/rw/RWB.NSF/db900SID/VBOL-6CQCQ2?OpenDocument

28. Levine, C. 1995. Today's challenges, tomorrow's dilemmas. In *Forgotten Children of the AIDS Epidemic,* ed. S.Geballe, J. Gruendel and W. Andiman. New Haven: Yale University Press.

29. Foster, G., C. Makufa, R. Drew, S. Kambeu and K. Saurombe. 1996. Supporting Children in Need through a Community-Based Orphan Visiting Program. *AIDS Care* 8:389-403.

30. Ibid 13.

Chapter 3

1. Africa's Orphaned Generations
http://www.unicef.org/publications/files/africas_orphans.pdf

2. *The National School Lunch Program Background and Development* Gordon W. Gunderson

http://www.fns.usda.gov/cnd/lunch/AboutLunch/ProgramHistory_2.htm

3. Africa's Orphaned Generations http://www.unicef.org/publications/files/africas_orphans.pdf
4. A Program on Orphans and Vulnerable Children in AIDS affected areas in Burkina Faso *Overview and Status Report.* http://www.axios-group.com
5. *400,000 AIDS Orphans In Mozambique*, Jan Lamprecht, *Southern Africa in Crisis* AfricanCrisis.org News24.com 11-7-3. http://www.rense.com/general44/mozab.htm
6. *We will Bury Ourselves* A Study of Child-Headed Households on Commercial Farms in Zimbabwe. http://www.synergyAIDS.com/documents/zimbabwe_children.pdf
7. AIDS Orphan Nutrition: a Question. http://www.unicef.org/publications/files/africas_orphans.pdf
8. MOZAMBIQUE: Mozambique Struggling to Feed Growing Number of AIDS Orphans, Associated Press (11.05.03) - Wednesday, November 05, 2003 Elliott Sylvester. http://www.aegis.com/news/ads/2003/AD032297.html

Chapter 4

1. *AIDS Orphans: Facing Africa's "Silent Crisis*, By Michael Fleshman, *Africa Recovery*, Vol.15 #3, October 2001, page 1. http://www.un.org/ecosocdev/geninfo/afrec/vol15no3/153child.htm
2. From a book review *of Children of AIDS: Africa's orphan crisis.* Emma Guest. http://www.iss.co.za/pubs/ASR/11No2/BookRev.html
3. Guest, Emma *Children of AIDS: Africa's Orphan Crisis.* 2003.
4. http://www.crin.org/
5. Gavan O'Sullivan, United Kingdom, Health/Medical Professional on 7/19/2004. http://qa.AIDSmatters.org/answer/10882

6. HIV/AIDS and Child Labour: A state-of-the-art review with recommendations for action Synthesis report by Bill Rau 2003. http://www.ilo.org/public/english/employment/gems/eeo/program/france/nfao.htm

7. Kenya's National Policy on Orphans and Vulnerable Children www.policyproject.com/pubs/generalreport/OVC_Policies.pdf

8. *We Will Bury Ourselves*, A Study of Child-Headed Households on Commercial Farms in Zimbabwe. http://www.synergyAIDS.com/documents/zimbabwe_children.pdf

9. Why are Girls Still Held Back? 2003/4. http://portal.unesco.org/education/en/ev.php-URL_ID=24156&URL_DO=DO_TOPIC&URL_SECTION=201.html

10. *HIV/AIDS and Food Security in Africa* A report for DFID Alex de Waal and Joseph Tumushabe 1 February 2003. http://www.sarpn.org.za/documents/d0001386/links.php

11. Helping AIDS orphans in childheaded households in Uganda http://www.crin.org/docs/resources/treaties/crc.40/GDD_2005_Plan_Finland.pdf

12. *The International Resilience Project: Findings from the Research and the Effectiveness of Interventions* Edith H. Grotberg, Ph.D., Senior Scientist, Civitan International Research Center, UAB 1997. http://resilnet.uiuc.edu/library/grotb97a.html

13. Africa's Youth on the Edge of the Chasm. Stephen Lewis raises alarm over loss of young women to HIV/AIDS. Africa Renewal, Vol.18 #3 (October 2004), page 9. http://www.un.org/ecosocdev/geninfo/afrec/vol18no3/183AIDS_lewis.htm

14. RESULTS Global Action Opportunities March 31, 2004. http://www.results.org/website/search.asp?topNavSearchInput=microenterprise

Chapter 5

1. AIDS Orphans: AIDS Orphans Set to Double by 2010. Agence France-Presse - July 10, 2002
Richard Ingham.
http://www.aegis.com/news/afp/2002/AF0207B5.html

2. From Single Parents to Child-Headed Households: the Case of Children Orphaned by AIDS in Kisumu and Siaya Districts, a research project report by Ayieko, mMA, Ph.D. 1997. http://www.undp.org/hiv/publications/study/english/sp7e.htm
3. Africa's Orphaned Generations http://www.unicef.org/publications/files/africas_orphans.pdf
4. Kalanidhi Subbarao and Diane Coury in *Reaching Out to Africa's Orphans: A Framework for Public Action* published by the World Bank in 2004. http://siteresources.worldbank.org/INTHIVAIDS/Resources/375798-1103037153392/ReachingOuttoAfricasOrphans.pdf
5. Introduction to AIDS in Zambia http://www.avert.org/AIDS-zambia.htm
6. Old Mutual Social Investment 2002. http://www2.oldmutual.com/CR/reports/ccr/2002/social/social_investment.asp
7. Melissa Fay Greene http://melissafaygreene.com/pages/afrAIDSorph.html
8. Child Sponsorships 2006. http://www.angelcovers.org/childsponsorship.html
9. The Children's Place Association http://www.childrens-place.org/
10. *Agencies to Help Children of HIV-Positive Parents* Divya Ramamurthi. http://www.hindu.com/2005/10/22/stories/2005102203340500.htm
11. Adoption from South Africa 2006 http://www.africasangels.org/AdoptionSouthAfrica.html
12. *A Generation of Orphans: Another Challenge for AIDS-Ravaged Countries* Laura Deame Editor: Wendy Vanasselt May 2001. http://earthtrends.wri.org/features/view_feature.php?theme=4&fid=22
13. *The Rise and Demise of the American Orphanage* Dale Keiger. http://www.jhu.edu/~jhumag/496web/orphange.html

14. Kalanidhi Subbarao and Diane Coury in *Reaching Out to Africa's Orphans: A Framework for Public Action* published by the World Bank in 2004.

http://siteresources.worldbank.org/INTHIVAIDS/Resources/375798-1103037153392/ReachingOuttoAfricasOrphans.pdf

15. *Second Home: Orphan Asylums and Poor Families in America* Timothy A. Hacsi, 1998.
http://www.amazon.com/gp/product/0674796446/

16. *The Home: A Memoir of Growing Up in an Orphanage* Richard McKenzie 1996.
http://www.alibris.com/search/search.cfm?qwork=2972096&wauth=Richard%20McKenzie&matches=14&qsort=r&cm_re=works*listing*title

17. *Community Care for Orphaned Children: What is Required?* L. Mudekunye & F. Napier. Save the Children UK, Pretoria, South Africa 2004.
http://www.iasociety.org/abstract/show.asp?abstract_id=2168280

18. AIDS Orphans: The Facts.
http://www.avert.org/AIDSorphans.htm

19. *A Generation of Orphans: Another Challenge for AIDS-Ravaged Countries* Laura Deame, Editor: Wendy Vanasselt. Date: May 2001.
http://earthtrends.wri.org/features/view_feature.php?theme=4&fid=22

20. Orphans and Vulnerable Children Reflecting on AIDS with Dr Mannasseh Phiri. 2005. http://kasisi.org/reflections_AIDS.html

21. Guiding Principles for Working with Orphans and Other Children Made Vulnerable by HIV/AIDS -The International Red Cross.

22. Orphans and other Children affected by HIV/AIDS
http://www.unicef.org/publications/pub_factsheet_orphan_en.pdf

23. Ibid 12

24. *Orphan Living Situations in Malawi: A Comparison of Orphanages and Foster Homes.* Ansell and Young, 2004 May 19, 2005 Brigitte Zimmerman. bazimm@stanford.edu

25. Kalanidhi Subbarao and Diane Coury in *Reaching Out to Africa's Orphans: Framework for Public Action* published by the World Bank in 2004. http://siteresources.worldbank.org/INTHIVAIDS/Resources/375798-1103037153392/ReachingOuttoAfricasOrphans.pdf
26. Child-Headed Households—AIDS Matters Questions and Answers http://qa.AIDSmatters.org/answer/10882/
27. Ibid 11
28. O'Sullivan, Gavan *Starting from Strengths. Social Exclusion, Rights Based Approach and Children in Charge of Families Affected by HIV/AIDS in Uganda.* Dissertation submitted to: London School of Economics and Political Science University of London. September, 2003.
29. African Charter on the Rights and Welfare of the Child, OAU Doc. CAB/LEG/24.9/49 (1990), *entered into force* Nov. 29, 1999. http://www1.umn.edu/humanrts/africa/afchild.htm
30. Children's Risk, Resilience, and Coping in Extreme Situations. Jo Boyden & Gillian Mann. 2005 in *Handbook for Working with Children and Youth Pathways to Resilience Across Cultures and Contexts* Authored by: Michael Ungar Dalhousie University. http://www.sagepub.co.uk/booksProdTOC.nav?prodId=Book226565
31. Children on the Brink 2004. http://pdf.dec.org/pdf_docs/PNACY333.pdf
32. Janet Museveni. http://www1.worldbank.org/sp/safetynets/OVCWorkshop_5-03/Orphans%20Analysis%20in%20Uganda.pdf

Chapter 6 - Conclusion

1. Encyclical Letter *Deus Caritas Est* of the Supreme Pontiff, Benedict XVI. http://www.vatican.va/holy_father/benedict_xvi/encyclicals/documents/hf_ben-xvi_enc_20051225_deus-caritas-est_en.html
2. Kofi Annan. 2001 Nobel Peace Prize. http://en.thinkexist.com/quotation/to_live_is_to_choose-but_to_choose_well-you_must/151784.html
3. Ibid 1

4. Message of His Holiness Pope John Paul II For the Celebration of the World Day of Peace 1 January 1996. Let us Give Children a Future of Peace. http://www.medjugorje.org/pope2.htm

For More Information

Journal Articles

Adhiambo Ogwang, E. (2001). Child Fostering in Kenya. From Care to Abuse. Paper presented at 12th Conference on Foster Care. International Foster Care Organization IFCO , Koningshof, Veldhoven, Netherlands, July 15–20.

Alden, J.S., G.M. Salole and J. Williamson. (1991). Managing Uganda's Orphan Crisis. Kampala: Technologies for Primary Health Care PRITECH Project.

Alliance. (2001). Expanding Community-Based Support for Orphans and Vulnerable Children. Family AIDS Caring Trust FACT and International HIV/AIDS Alliance.

Ansell & Young. (2004) Orphan Living Situations in Malawi: A Comparison of Orphanages and Foster Homes May 19, 2005 Brigitte Zimmerman bazimm@stanford.edu

Arvidson, M. (1996). Caring for Children: Orphans in the AIDS-Affected in Zimbabwe. *Program on Population and Development, Report No. 13.* Lund, Sweden: University of Lund.

Ayieko, M. A. (1997). From Single Parents to Child-Headed Households: The Case of Children Orphaned by AIDS in Kisumu and Siaya Districts. Study Paper No. 7. University of Illinois, Dept. of International Programs and Studies. New York: United Nations Development Programme.

Aspaas, H. R. (1999). AIDS and Orphans in Uganda: Geographical and Gender Interpretation of Household Resources. *Social Science Journal* 36 2: 201–226.

Bandawe, C. R., and Louw, J. (1997). The Experience of Family Foster Care in Malawi: A Preliminary Investigation. *Child Welfare* 86 July/August :535–547.

Barrett, K. (1998). The Right of Children: Raising the Orphan Generation. Paper presented at *Conference on Raising the Orphan Generation*, organized by CINDI, Children in Distress, Pietermaritzburg, June 9–12.

Barnett, T., & Blaikie, P. (1992). The Special Case of Orphans. In *AIDS in Africa: Present and future impact* pp. 110-126. London: Belhaven Press.

Basaza, R., & Kaija, D. (2002). The Impact of HIV/AIDS on Children: Lights and Shadows in the "Successful Case" of Uganda. In G. A. Cornia Ed., *AIDS, public policy and child well-being.* Florence, Italy: United Nations Children's Fund.

Beers, C., et. al. (1996). AIDS: The Grandmother's Burden. In *The Global Impact of AIDS*, eds. A. F. Fleming and others. New York: Liss.

Bhargava, A. and Bigombe, B. (2003). Public Policies and the Orphans of AIDS in Africa. *British Medical Journal, v. 326, no. 7403,* p. 1387-89.

Bicego, G; Rutstein, S. and Johnson, K. (2003). Dimensions of the Emerging Orphan Crisis in Sub-Saharan Africa. *Social Science & Medicine, v. 56, no. 6,* p. 1235-1247.

Bikini, S.S. (1999). Children in Residential Care Prevention Social Policy Strategy: The Ugandan experience.

Bledsoe, C.H., Ewbank, D.C. and Isiugo-Abanihe, U.C. (1988). The Effect of Child Fostering on Feeding Practices and Access to Health Services in Rural Sierra Leone. *Social Science and Medicine* 27 (6): 627–636.

Brink, P. (1998). Adoption Practice in the AIDS Era. A South African Perspective. Paper presented at *Conference on Raising the Orphan Generation*, organized by CINDI (Children in Distress), Pietermaritzburg, June 9–12.

Bukenya, S.S. (1999), April. Children in Residential Care Prevention: Social policy strategy. The Uganda Experience. Kampala, Uganda: Ministry of Gender, Labour and Social Development, Department of Childcare and Protection.

Chernet, T. (2001). Overview of Services for Orphans and Vulnerable Children in Ethiopia. Report version of presentation at national workshop, Kigali, Rwanda, March 27–29, 2001. April 26.

Community Members Concerning the Circumstances of Orphans in Rural Zimbabwe. *AIDS Care* 9: 391–406.

Connolly, M. (2001). Principles to Guide Programming for Orphans and Other Vulnerable Children Affected by HIV/AIDS. Draft, United Nations Children's Fund UNICEF, New York.

Connolly, M., Lorey, M., Mahalingam, M., Sussman, L., & Williamson, J. (2000). *Principles to Guide Programming for Orphans and Other Vulnerable Children.* New York: UNICEF

Dane, O. B., & Levine, C. (1994). *AIDS and the New Orphans: Coping with Death.* Westport, CT: Auborn House.

Dansky, S.F. (1997). *Nobody's Children: Orphans of the HIV epidemic.* New York: Harrington Park Press.

Deininger, K., Garcia, M., and Subbarao, K. (2003). AIDS-Induced Orphans as Systemic Shock: Magnitude, Impact and Program Interventions in Africa. *World Development* 31 (7): 1201–1220.

Desmond, C. (2002). The Economic Evaluation of Models of Care for Orphaned and Vulnerable Children. Paper prepared for Family Health International, Research Triangle Park, NC.

Desmond, C., and Gow, J. (2001). The Cost-Effectiveness of 6 Models of Care for Orphans and Other Vulnerable Children. Health Economics and HIV/AIDS Research HEARD, University of Natal and UNICEF, Durban, South Africa

Drew, R, Makufa, C. and Foster, G. (1998). Strategies for Providing Care and Support to Children Orphaned by AIDS. *AIDS Care-Psychological and Socio-Medical Aspects of AIDS/HIV, v. 10, no. 1,* p. 9-15.

Dunn, A., Hunter, S., Nabongo, C., & Sekiwanuka, J. (1991). Enumeration and Needs Assessment of Orphans in Uganda: A Survey Report. Kampala, Uganda: Makerere University, Department of Sociology.

Foster, G., R. Shakespeare, F. Chinemana, C. Makufa & Drew. R. (1995). Orphan Prevalence and Extended Family Care in a Peri-Urban Community in Zimbabwe. *AIDS Care* 7:3-17.

Foster, G., Makufa, C. and R. Drew. (1995). Am I My Brother's Keeper? Orphans, AIDS and the Extended Family's Choice of Caregiver. *Sociétés d'Afrique and SIDA Newsletter,* October. Bordeaux.

Foster, G., C. Makufa, R. Drew, S. Kambeu and K. Saurombe. 1996. Supporting Children in Need through a Community-Based Orphan Visiting Program. *AIDS Care* 8:389-403.

Foster, G., Makufa, C., Drew, R., Mashumba, S., & Kambeu S. (1997). Perceptions of Children and Community Members Concerning the Circumstances of Orphans in Rural Zimbabwe. *AIDS Care* 9: 393-407.

Foster G., C. Makufa, R. Drew, & E. Kralovec. (1997a). Factors Leading to the Establishment of Child-Headed Households: The Case of Zimbabwe. *Health Transition Review* supplement 2,7: 155–168.

Foster G., C. Makufa, R. Drew, et. al. (1997b). Perceptions of Children and Government of Zambia. 1999. Situation Analysis of Orphans in Zambia, 1999. A Joint USAIS/UNICEF/SIDA Study, Lusaka.

Foster, G. (2000). Responses in Zimbabwe to Children Affected by AIDS. *SAfAIDS News* 8 (1).

Foster G., and J. Williamson. (2000). A Review of Current Literature of the Impact of HIV/AIDS on Children in Sub-Saharan Africa. *AIDS 2000* 14 supplement 3: S275–284.

Foster, G. (2002). Supporting Community Efforts to Assist Orphans in Africa. *New England Journal of Medicine, v. 346, no. 24,* p. 1907-10. Foster, G. 1997. "Orphans." *AIDS Care – Psychological and Socio-Medical Aspects of AIDS/HIV, v. 9, no. 1,* p. 82-87.

Gregson, S., Garnett, G.P., & Anderson, R.M. (1994). Assessing the Potential Impact of the HIV-1 Epidemic on Orphanhood and the Demographic Structure of Populations in Sub-Saharan Africa. *Population Studies* 48: 435–458.

Grodney, D. (1994). Programs for Children and Adolescents. In *AIDS and the New Orphans*, ed. B. O. Dane and C. Levine. Westport: Auburn House.

Halkett, R. (1998). *Enhancing the Quality of Life for Children without Parents in the South African Context* Paper presented at Conference on Raising the Orphan Generation, organized by CINDI, Pietermaritzburg, June 9–12.

Harber, M. (1998). *Developing a Community-Based AIDS Orphan Project. A South African Case Study* Paper presented at Conference on Raising the Orphan Generation, organized by CINDI, Pietermaritzburg, June 9–12.

Harrison, K., Sophal, L.C., & Edström., J. (2001). Supporting Non-governmental Organizations to Develop Locally Appropriate Indicators for Work with Orphans and Vulnerable Children.

Hunter, S. (1990). Orphans as a Window on the AIDS Epidemic in Sub-Saharan Africa: Initial Results and Implications of a Study in Uganda. *Social Science and Medicine*, 31 (6), 681-690.

Hunter, S. & Williamson, J. (1997) Children on the Brink. Strategies to Support Children Isolated by HIV/AIDS. Arlington, VA. Health Technical Services Project of Associates and the Pragma Corporation for the HIV/AIDS Division of U.S. Agency for International Development USAID.

Hunter, S. & Williamson, J. (2000). Children on the Brink: Strategies to Support Children Isolated by HIV/AIDS. Arlington, VA: USAID.

Kalemba, E. (1998). *The Development of an Orphans Policy and Programming in Malawi* Paper presented at Conference on Raising the Orphan Generation, organized by CINDI, Pietermaritzburg, June 9–12.

Kamali, A., Seeley, J.A., Nunn, A.J., Kengeya-Kayondo, J.F., Ruberantwari, A. & Mulder, D.W. (1996). The Orphan Problem: Experience of a Sub-Saharan Africa Rural Population in the AIDS Epidemic. *AIDS Care*, Vol. 8, No. 5, October 1996, pp. 509 - 516

Krift, T., and Phiri, S. (1998). Developing a Strategy to Strengthen Community Capacity to Assist HIV/AIDS-Affected Children and Families: The COPE Program of Save the Children Federation in Malawi. Paper presented at Conference on Raising the Orphan Generation, Pietermaritzburg, June 9–12.

Landgren, K. (1998), October 27. Rights-Based Approach to the Care and Protection of Orphans. United Nations Children's Fund.

Levine, C. (1995.) Today's challenges, tomorrow's dilemmas. In *Forgotten Children of the AIDS Epidemic*, ed. S.Geballe, J. Gruendel and W. Andiman. New Haven: Yale University Press.

Lightfoot, M. and Rotheram-Borus, M. (2004). Predictors of Child Custody Plans for Children Whose Parents Are Living with AIDS in New York City. *Social Work*, Vol. 49, 2004.

Linsk, N.L. (2004). Stresses on Grandparents and Other Relatives Caring for Children Affected by HIV/AIDS Journal article by Nathan L. Linsk, Sally Mason; *Health and Social Work*, Vol. 29,

Lucas C & Harber M 1997. Evaluation of the Valley Trust HIV/AIDS Programme: The Ithemba Ngekusasa - Hope For the Future- AIDS Programme. Centre for Health and Social Studies, University of Natal, Durban.

MacLeod, H. 2001. Residential Care. In *Orphans and Other Vulnerable Children: What Role for Social Protection?* ed. A. Levine. Proceedings for World Bank/World Vision Conference, June 6–7.

Masmas, T. N; Jensen, H; da Silva, D; Hoj, L; Sandstrom, A. and Aaby, P. 2004. The Social Situation of Motherless Children in Rural and Urban Areas of Guinea-Bissau. *Social Science & Medicine, v. 59,* p. 1231-1239.

Mbugua, T. (2004) Responding to the Special Needs of Children: Educating HIV/AIDS Orphans in Kenya; *Childhood Education*, Vol. 80.

Michaels, D. 1994. Projections of Motherless AIDS Orphans under 15 in Six Countries. In *Action for Children Affected by AIDS - Programme Profiles and Lessons Learned.* New York: World Health Organization/UNICEF.

Monk, N. 2001. Underestimating the magnitude of a mature crisis: Dynamics of Orphaning and Fostering in Rural Uganda. Orphan Alert: International Perspectives on Children Left Behind by HIV/AIDS. New York.

Mukoyogo, M C & Williams G. 1991. AIDS Orphans, A Community Perspective from Tanzania. Strategies for Hope Series. Action Aid/AMFREF/World in Need UNICEF 1991 AIDS and Orphans in Africa. Conference Report, Florence 14th-15th June 1991. New York, UNICEF.

Muller, O., & Abbas, N. 1990. The Impact of AIDS Mortality on Children's Education in Kampala. AIDS Care, 2(1), 77-80.

Muller, O., Sen, G., & Nsubuga, A. (1999). HIV/AIDS, Orphans and Access to School Education in a Community of Kampala, Uganda. *AIDS Care*, 13(1), 146-147.

National Council for Children. (1999). Uganda's Commitment to Children by the End of the Century: A Report on the Implementation of the UN Convention on the Rights of the Child from 1990 to 1999.

Neema, S. et al. (2000). Children Living in Difficult Circumstances: Vulnerability and Coping Mechanisms of Child-Headed Households in Rakai, Uganda. Lutheran World Federation, Department of World Service, Uganda Programme, Rakai Project & Makerere Institute for Social Research.

Ntambirweki, P. 2001. *Assessment of the Orphan Situation in Bundibugyo District* Report. Uganda

Ntozi, J. P. et al. 1995. Care for AIDS Orphans in Uganda: Findings from Focus Group Discussions. *Health Transition Review*, 5 Supplement, 245-252.

Ntozi, J.P., Ahimbisibwe, F.E., Odwee, J.O., Ayiga, N. & Okurut, F.N. 1999. Orphan Care: the Role of the Extended Family in Northern Uganda. In *The Continuing HIV/AIDS Epidemic in Africa: Responses and Coping Strategies*. I.O. Orubuloye, J. Caldwell & J. P. Ntozi, eds. Canberra: Health Transition Centre, pp.225-236.

Nyambedha, EO, Wandibba, S. & Aagaard-Hansen, J. 2001. Policy Implications of the Inadequate Support Systems for Orphans in Western Kenya. *Health Policy*, 58, 83-96.

Nyambedha, EO, Wandibba, S. & Aagaard-Hansen, J. (2003). Changing Patterns of Orphan Care Due to the HIV Epidemic in Western Kenya. *Social Science & Medicine* 57 (2003) 301-311.

O'Sullivan, Gavan *Starting from Strengths. Social Exclusion, Rights Based Approach and Children in Charge of Families Affected by HIV/AIDS in Uganda.* Dissertation submitted to: London School of Economics and Political Science University of London. September, 2003.

Panpanich, R., Brabin, B., Gonani, A., & Graham, S. 1999. Are Orphans at Increased Risk of Malnutrition in Malawi? *Annals of Tropical Paediatrics*, 3, 279-285.

Poonawala, S. & Cantor, R. 1991. Children orphaned by AIDS: A call for Action for NGOS and Donors. Washington, DC: National Council for International Health.

Rutayuga, J. 1992. Assistance to AIDS Orphans within the Family Kinship System and Local Institutions – A Program for East-Africa. *AIDS Education and Prevention, supplement*, p. 57-68.

Ryder, RW; Kamenga, M; Nkusu, M; Batter, V. and Heyward, W. 1994. "AIDS Orphans in Kinhasa, Zaire – Incidence and Socio-economic Consequences." *AIDS*, v. 8, no. 5, p. 673-679.

Salaam, T. 2004. AIDS Orphans and Vulnerable Children: Problems, Responses and Issues for Congress. *Congressional Research Service*. The Library of Congress.

Saoke, P. & Mutemi, R. 1996. Needs Assessment of Children Orphaned by AIDS: Nairobi: UNICEF Country office.

Saoke, P., R. Mutemi and C. Blair. 1996. Another Song Begins: Children Orphaned by AIDS. Pp. 45-64 in *AIDS in Kenya: Socio-economic Impact and Policy Implications*, ed. S. Forsythe and B. Rau. Arlington: Family Health International/ AIDSCAP.

Schoenteich, M. 2001. *A Generation at Risk: AIDS Orphans, Vulnerable Children and Human Security in Africa* Paper presented at Conference on Orphans and Vulnerable Children in Africa, convened by the Nordic Africa Institute and the Danish Bilharziasis Laboratory. Uppsala, September 13–16.

Sengendo, J., and J. Nambi. 1997. The Psychological Effect of Orphanhood: A Study of Orphans in Rakai District. *Health Transition Review* supplement 105–124.

Siaens, C., K. Subbarao, and Q. T. Wodon. 2003. Are Orphans Especially Vulnerable? Evidence from Rwanda. World Bank, Washington, DC.

Subbarao K., A. Mattimore, and K. Plangemann. 2001. Social Protection of Africa's Orphans and Other Vulnerable Children. *Issues and Good Practices: Program Options*. Africa Region, Human Development Working Paper Series, World Bank, Washington, DC.

Suda, C. 1997. Street Children in Nairobi and the African ideology of Kin-Based Support Systems. *Child Abuse Review*, 6, 199-217.

Uganda Foster Care and Adoption Association UFCAA. 1994 . Uganda's 50-Year Experience in Child Adoption: A Study of Applicants at the Uganda High Court, 1943-1993. Kampala, Uganda: Uganda Foster Care and Adoption Association Publications.

UNAIDS and UNICEF launch the *Children in a World with AIDS* Initiative. Factsheet. 28 August. Stockholm.

United Nations Children's Fund. 1999. Orphans and Vulnerable Children: A Situation Analysis of Orphans in Zambia, 1999. New York, NY.

United Nations Children's Fund-Zambia. (2000). Eastern and Southern Africa Regional Workshop on Orphans and Vulnerable Children. Workshop report, November 5-8. Lusaka, Zambia.

United Nations Children's Fund-Uganda. (2001). Realising the Rights of Children Affected and Orphaned by HIV/AIDS - Donor proposal, Executive Summary, p. 4. New York.

United Nations Children's Fund. (2001). Ten years after: Celebrating Uganda's Success in Implementing Children's Rights.

Urassa, M., J.T. Boerma, J Z.L. Ng'weshemi, R. Isingo, D. Shapink, and Y. Kumogola. 1997. Orphanhood, Child Fostering and the AIDS Epidemic in Rural Tanzania. *Health Transition Review* (supplement 2) 7: 41–153.

Wane, N. N. & Kavuma, E. (2001). "Grandmothers Called out of Retirement: The Challenges for African Women Facing AIDS Today." *Canadian Woman Studies Journal.* 21 (2): 10-19.

Webb, D. 1995. Who Will Take Care of the AIDS Orphans? *AIDS Analysis Africa* 5(2): 12–13.

Williamson, J. 1995. Children and Families Affected by HIV/AIDS: Guidelines for Action Report.

Washington DC: Displaced Children and Orphans Fund and War Victims Fund of USAID.

Williamson, J. 2000a. Finding a Way Forward: Principles and Strategies to Reduce the Impacts of AIDS on Children and Families. Displaced Children and Orphans Fund and War Victims Fund Contract, U.S. Agency for International Development, Washington, DC, March.

Wolff, P. and Fesseha, G. 1998. "The Orphans of Eritrea: Are Orphanages Part of the Problem or Part of the Solution?" *American Journal of Psychiatry,* v. 15, no. 10, p. 1319-1324.

World Health Organisation, Global Programme on AIDS. 1995. The Role of the Committee on the Rights of the Child and its Impact on HIV/AIDS: Problems and Prospects. Presentation at AIDS and Child Rights: The Impact of the Asia-Pacific Region, Bangkok, Thailand, 21-26 November.

Books

Best, J. (1994). A Threatened Generation: Impediments to Children's Quality of Life in Kenya in *Troubling Children: Studies of Children and Social Problems*. Aldine De Gruyter: New York.

Books, S. (1998). The Crisis within the Crisis: The Growing Epidemic of AIDS Orphans in *Invisible Children in the Society and Its Schools.*: Mahwah, NJ: Lawrence Erlbaum Associates.

Dane & Levine (1994). *AIDS and the New Orphans: Coping with Death*. Auburn House Paperback, 1994.

Greene, M.F. (2006) *There Is No Me Without You: One Woman's Odyssey to Rescue Africa's Children*. Bloomsbury Publishing PLC.

Guest, E. (2003). *Children of AIDS: Africa's Orphan Crisis, 2nd Ed.* Pluto Press.

Joslin, D. (2002). *Invisible Caregivers: Older Adults Raising Children in the Wake of HIV/AIDS*. Columbia University Press.

LeVack, D. (2005). *God's Golden Acre: The Inspirational Story of One Woman's Fight for Some of the World's Most Vulnerable AIDS Orphan*. Monarch Books.

Sills, Y.G. (1994). *The AIDS Pandemic: Social Perspectives*. Greenwood Press.

Williamson, J., et. al. (2005). *A Generation at Risk: The Global Impact of HIV/AIDS on Orphans and Vulnerable Children*. Cambridge University Press.

Electronic References

(sorted by year, as available)

Pediatric AIDS Now Considered a Global Threat; Millions Expected to Become Orphans Magazine article by Anne-Christine D'Adesky; UN Chronicle, Vol. 27, December 1990. http://www.thefreelibrary.com/Pediatric+AIDS+now+considered+a+global+threat%3B+millions+expected+to...-a09280940

AIDS orphans: Africa's lost generation. AIDS claims the lives of several parents in Africa: An article from: World Watch [HTML] Aaron Sachs, September 1, 1993.

http://www.thefreelibrary.com/AIDS+orphans:+Africa's+lost+generation-a014538624

Qualitative Needs Assessment of Child-Headed Households in Rwanda, by World Vision with support from UNICEF. January 1998. http://www.epals.com/waraffectedchildren/chap4/

Berret, K. 2000. The rights of children: Raising the orphan generation [Data file]. http://www/togan.co.za/cindi/papers/paper11.htm

Of AIDS Orphans and Party Pigs. Brendon Lemon; The Advocate, February 29, 2000. http://findarticles.com/p/articles/mi_m1589/is_2000_Feb_29/ai_59587052

Joint United Nations Programme on HIV/AIDS. UNAIDS. 1999. Children orphaned by AIDS: Front-line responses from eastern and southern Africa. Geneva, Switzerland: Joint United Nations Programme on HIV/AIDS. http://www.unAIDS.org/publications/documents/children/

United Nations Children's Fund-Tanzania. 1999. Children in need of special protection measures. A Tanzania study. Accessed May 2002. www.unicef.org/cap/CAPall.pdf

International Obligation and Human Health: Evolving Policy Responses to HIV/AIDS Paul G. Harris, Patricia Siplon; Ethics & International Affairs, Vol. 15, 2001. http://www.healthgap.org/press_releases/05/2001_Siplon_article_international_obligation.html

AIDS orphans and vulnerable children in Africa: Identifying the best practices for care, treatment, and prevention: hearing, tenth Congress, second session, April 17, 2002 http://www.communitylawcentre.org.za/ser/esr2002/2002july_child.php

The growth of AIDS orphans and policy solutions. Legislative and Policy Update. *Pediatric Nursing* [HTML] Eileen Meier. January 1, 2003. http://goliath.ecnext.com/coms2/gi_0199-2510201/The-growth-of-AIDS-orphans.html

A Pilgrim's Progress: Metaphor in the Rhetoric of Mary Fisher, AIDS Activist Jennifer J. Mcgee; *Women's Studies in Communication*, Vol. 26, 2003.

http://www.accessmylibrary.com/coms2/summary_0286-2310988_ITM

Congregation helps Ugandan AIDS orphans: a small, caring organization does what it can for a huge, devastating problem. Canadian news: An article from: Presbyterian Record [HTML] Tom Dickey 2003
http://findarticles.com/p/articles/mi_go2566/is_200309/ai_n9247641

A review of current literature of the impact of HIV/AIDS on children in sub-Saharan Africa By: USA Agency for International Development USAID Source: Eldis Date: 2003-10-21
http://www.africapulse.org.za/index.php?action=viewarticle&articleid=1661

Kalanidhi Subbarao and Diane Coury in Reaching Out to Africa's Orphans: A Framework for Public Action published by the World Bank in 2004.
http://siteresources.worldbank.org/INTHIVAIDS/Resources/375798-1103037153392/ReachingOuttoAfricasOrphans.pdf

AIDS Leaves Heavy Burden on Orphans; Support Collapses for Millions. The Washington Times, February 19, 2004.
http://goliath.ecnext.com/coms2/gi_0199-2367472/AIDS-leaves-heavy-burden-on.html

AIDS Orphans and Vulnerable Children OVC: problems, responses, and issues for congress. : An article from: Congressional Research Service CRS Reports and Issue Briefs [HTML] Tiaji Salaam March 1, 2004.
http://usinfo.state.gov/gi/img/assets/5096/rl32252102605.pdf

Number of AIDS Orphans to Skyrocket in 6 Years, Study Says *The Washington Times*, March 9, 2004.
http://www.thebody.com/content/art26477.html

No Schools for Orphans as Mugabe Pours Cash into Arms David Blair; *Daily Telegraph London*, England , June 23, 2004.
http://www.telegraph.co.uk/news/main.jhtml;?xml=/news/2004/06/23/wzim23.xml

Responding to the special needs of children: educating HIV/AIDS orphans in Kenya Childhood Education [HTML] Tata Mbugua

August 15, 2004.
http://www.eric.ed.gov/ERICWebPortal/recordDetail?accno=EJ705756

AIDS Orphans: When You Die, How Should I Do This? Magazine article by Oksana Kim; UN Chronicle, Vol. 41, June 2004.
http://findarticles.com/p/articles/mi_m1309/is_2_41/ai_n6232048

The AIDS Orphans of South Africa, in *Contemporary* Review Carol Landman. 3 pgs.
http://findarticles.com/p/articles/mi_m2242/is_1642_281/ai_94775536

Children of Conflict: Child Headed Households
http://www.bbc.co.uk/worldservice/people/features/childrensrights/childrenofconflict/headed.shtml

HIV and AIDS in Africa. http://www.avert.org/aidsinafrica.htm

Children At Risk http://www.viva.org/?page_id=8risks.php

Mothers Without Borders. http://www.motherswithoutborders.org

A Ray of Hope for Orphans in Zambia.
http://www.hopeforAIDS.org/story.asp?id=29

African Orphans. http://www.africanorphans.com/

Children Taking on More Than They Can Handle.
http://www.prb.org/pdf/AIDSorphan.pdf

South Africa: Open School Project.
http://www.acsi.org/web2003/default.aspx?ID=2455

AIDS/HIV Statistics. http://www.avert.org/statindx.htm

"We will Bury Ourselves" *A Study of Child-Headed Households on Commercial Farms in Zimbabwe* Farm Orphan Support Trust of Zimbabwe Compiled by: Lynn Walker, Executive Director, FOST http://www.synergyAIDS.com/documents/zimbabwe_children.pdf

Adoption Advocates International.
http://www.adoptionadvocates.org/

New York Council on Adoptable Children. http://www.coac.org/

Adoption Resources. http://www.orphandoctor.com/adoption/

Ohio Adoption Information. http://www.adoptioninformation.com/

Pathfinder International http://www.pathfind.org/

From single parents to child-headed households: the case of children orphaned by AIDS in Kisumu and Siaya districts A research project report. Ayieko, M A, PHD http://www.undp.org/hiv/publications/study/English/sp7e.htm

Orphans and vulnerable children, early child development. World Bank http://www.worldbank.org/children/

Displaced Children and Orphans Fund (DCOF) http://www.usaid.gov/our_work/humanitarian_assistance/the_funds/dcof/index.html

Association François-Xavier Bagnoud http://www.orphans.fxb.org

Acknowledgements

This work could not have been completed without the support and generosity of the following people. With gratitude and prayers I thank...

Sr. Mary De Bacco, MPF, Superior General of the Religious Teachers Filippini

Sr. Ascenza Tizzano, MPF, Provincial Superior Religious Teachers Filippini USA

The Religious Teachers Filippini of Ethiopia, Eritrea, India, Brazil and Albania, Italy Ireland, England, Switzerland and the USA

Sr. Margherita Marchione, M.P.F.
Anita Branch
Gregory and Kathy Johnson
David McIntee
Jillian Coleman Wheeler
Christine Burrows Yi, MD
William Lloyd, MD
Maureen Lloyd
Joe Vitale
Lisa Smith-Batchen
Angelo D'Amelio
Andrea Schaeffer
Lianne Latkany
Rachel Barcia Morse
Noel and Virginia George
Lisa Lanterman
Suzanne Burns
Joseph Lunzer
Victor R. Volkman

About the Author

Sr. Mary Elizabeth Lloyd has been helping the orphans and the Child Headed Households of the missions of the Religious Teachers Filippini for the past 12 years. Her experiences in Albania, Brazil, Ethiopia, Eritrea and India have spurred her on to produce this work. Sister holds a doctorate degree in Nutrition and Public Health from Columbia University.

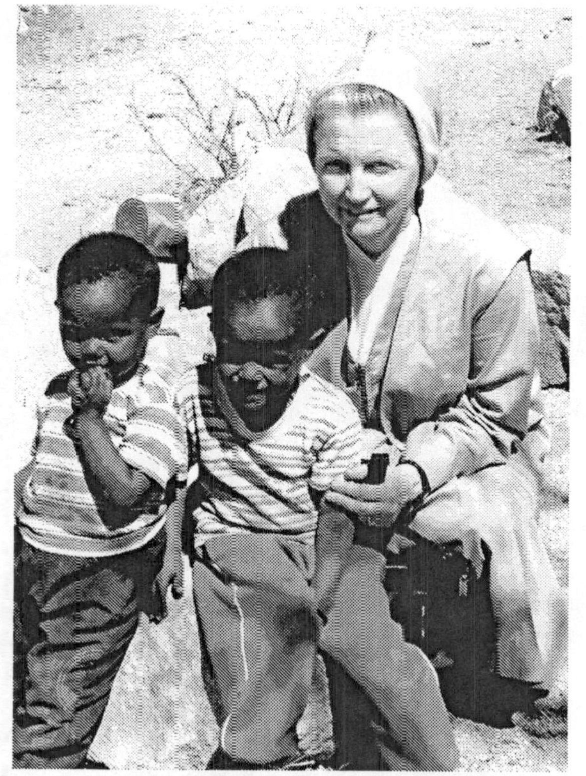

Pic. A-1: Sister Mary Elizabeth Lloyd with AIDS orphans

Religious Teachers Filippini

The Religious Teachers Filippini have been helping the poorest children and women survive for more than 300 years. In the past our schools and initiatives for orphans and widows were mainly due to the consequences of war. Now the times are changing and we are adapting by providing these same survival and life skills to the CHH. Many of our graduates have gone on to set up their own restaurants or sewing shops and others have gone on to be successful in business and technology, or as teachers and nurses.

It is very touching to see the former graduates return with their own families to thank the Sisters for all they have done for them. One very memorable event was when one of our former students returned with 500 eggs for the Sisters to use with the children. He recounted how he and his brother were starving when the Sisters took them in and not only fed them but loved, educated and provided for their every need. For more information about the Religious Teachers Filippin's work in the United States, please visit: www.filippiniusa.org

How Donations Make A Difference

The Religious Teachers Filippini will help you decide how you can help these children and make sure that 100% of your gift helps the CHH. You are also afforded the opportunity to visit and stay with the children so you can see how they are succeeding.

The CHH where the oldest member is over 12 is provided a small home, and enters a program where they learn a trade so they can earn some money right away for their little family, while also studying for their elementary education diploma. They learn sewing, knitting, embroidering, gardening, poultry raising. And are taught basic business skills to help their micro-enterprise be successful. The Religious Teachers will soon be opening a similar initiative for these children in Addis Abbab.

For all donations, please make checks payable to Religious Teachers Filippini and mail to:

Sr. Mary Beth Lloyd, MPF
Villa Walsh
455 Western Ave.
Morristown, NJ 07960

The Religious Teachers Filippini is a 5013(c) tax-deductible organization

Index

I

J

K

L

M

N

O

P

R

S

T